# 101 MIRACLE FOODS THAT HEAL YOUR HEART

## Liz Applegate, Ph.D.

Foreword by Paul D. Thompson, M.D.

PRENTICE HALL PRESS

**Library of Congress Cataloging-in-Publication Data**

Applegate, Elizabeth Ann.
   101 miracle foods that heal your heart / by Liz Applegate.
       p.  cm.
   Includes index.
   ISBN 0-7352-0169-2 (pbk.)
       1. Heart—Diseases—Diet therapy. 2. Heart—Diseases—Prevention.
   I. Title: One hundred and one miracle foods that heal your heart.
II. Title.
   RC684.D5 A66  2000
   616.1'20654—dc21

                                                              00-035678

© 2000 by Prentice Hall

Printed in the United States of America

10 9 8 7 6 5 4 3 2 1

ISBN 0-7352-0169-2

*This book is intended as a reference guide only, not as a medical manual to self-treatment. If you suspect that you have a medical problem, seek competent help. The information presented in this book is intended to help you make informed decisions about your diet, not to substitute for any treatment that may have been prescribed by your physician.*

---

ATTENTION: CORPORATIONS AND SCHOOLS
Prentice Hall books are available at quantity discounts with bulk purchase for educational, business, or sales promotional use. For information, please write to: Prentice Hall Special Sales, 240 Frisch Court, Paramus, New Jersey 07652. Please supply: title of book, ISBN, quantity, how the book will be used, date needed.

---

**PRENTICE HALL PRESS**
Paramus, NJ 07652

On the World Wide Web at http://www.phdirect.com

In memory of my father, Dr. Paul Kirk

# Acknowledgments

Many people gave from their heart in support of this book. I would like to thank my family—my husband, Mark, and my two children, Grant and Natalie—for their love and support not to mention willingness to try my new recipes. My thanks to Marlia Braun for her wonderful assistance in research and technical help; and thanks also to Jana Gonsalves for her nutrition expertise in analyzing the recipes and menus. And many thanks to chef Mumulay Rajan for her culinary advice, recipes, and ideas, as well as Ellen Moratti for her food and recipe suggestions. And finally to Terry, Ann, and Raul for their heart-warming friendship.

# Contents

## Chapter Two

## Chapter Three

# PART TWO

## Abalone to Zucchini:
## 101 Miracle Foods That Fit in the Simple Six
## 47

# Foreword

My full-time business is heart health. During my 20 years of practice I have worked with thousands of people trying to prevent heart disease and thousands more trying to prevent further damage after suffering from a heart attack or a stroke. Preventing heart disease is not easy and involves many factors, but I am convinced that what we eat has a major role in reducing such heart- and blood-vessel disease risk factors as high cholesterol levels, high blood pressure, obesity, and diabetes. Many patients incorrectly assume that the medicines their doctor prescribes to treat high cholesterol, diabetes, and hypertension are all that's needed. Unfortunately I often have to remind my patients that they "can eat their way through even the best medicines," meaning that a bad diet can undermine the most careful medical plan.

I am also convinced that people seeking the holy grail of a healthy heart need easy-to-understand and useful information about food. *101 Miracle Foods That Heal Your Heart* by my good friend, Liz Applegate, Ph.D., is certainly what this doctor ordered.

In the first part of her book, Dr. Applegate presents up-to-date information on the connection between heart disease and food. Such basic knowledge is critical for patients to know how to take care of themselves. Futher on, Liz reveals her "Simple Six Eating Plan," which is just that, simple. Anyone seeking to prevent heart disease can benefit from this healthful eating plan without making their diet a chore. I am pleased that soy is deliciously incorporated into the Simple Six Eating Plan. The full story on soy is still evolving, but soy appears to lower cholesterol levels and have other important health benefits as well. Liz has convinced me that I don't have to fly to Japan or even visit my local Benihana in order to enjoy the benefits of an oriental eating plan.

In the second part of her book, Dr. Applegate presents 101 foods that fit her Simple Six Eating Plan. For each food from apples to zucchini, she describes its nutritional profile and summarizes the research as to how the food may be beneficial for heart health. I was relieved to see that even chocolate, one of my favorites, has some redeeming values that allow it to play a role in a healthy diet. Liz also provides shopping, preparation, and cooking tips for each food along with great recipes.

Dr. Applegate has written over 300 articles on nutrition, health, and performance. I know how extensively she researches her work, and this book reflects that care by presenting the most current research on the food-heart health connection. But Liz also brings a unique perspective derived from her diverse background as an accomplished triathlete, a popular professor at the University of California, and the former director of a cardiac rehab program. With that sort of resumé, Liz has had experience working with all sorts of people, including, I'll bet, someone just like you.

From cover to cover, this book is packed with practical information for anyone wanting a healthy heart. Don't allow yourself ten years hence to say, "Would I be healthy if I had eaten right?" Avoid the "what ifs" and take steps now to protect and keep your heart healthy for the rest of your life.

Paul D. Thompson, M.D.
Professor of Medicine, University of Connecticut
Director of Preventive Cardiology, Hartford Hospital

*part one* ———————————

# Your Personal Plan
# to a Healthy Heart

# CHAPTER ONE

# *You and Your Heart*

Picture the scenario: You gobble down a whopping hot dog at the ball park. Or perhaps, you're out with a friend and you "splurge" with an extravagant, not to mention fatty, dinner and follow it with an even more sinfully fatty (but delicious) dessert. The fat zooms straight for your arteries, right? You worry that glob of fat may block off a blood vessel and you may collapse from a heart attack. You can almost feel it.

Well, not exactly. Certainly fat is dangerous for your heart, but how heart disease, stroke, and other diseases of the vascular system take hold is another story and one you'll want to know so you can hedge off disaster. An artery becomes lined with a cholesterol-fat buildup called plaque through a series of steps. Interrupting those steps, or at least delaying one or two, will give you an edge on heart health. Also, understanding what high blood pressure is and how you can control it with diet can keep this killer from creeping up on you.

Trust me, if you know how arteries become plugged in the first place, you're more apt to take action now. Scientists have unraveled the dark secrets of heart disease, much of which was a mystery until recently. The heart-disease story is actually quite simple and is a lot like a freeway system that has gone awry during rush hour.

## Unclogging the Myths About Heart Disease

Picture a large city with thousands of homes and businesses all in need of constant supplies—food, clothing, other provisions—everything to build and maintain this thriving mass of activity. Now let's say all those supplies come by truck into the city on a busy freeway. Unfortunately, over the years cars, trucks, and buses have been throwing their trash out their windows clogging the outer lanes of traffic with garbage. As a result, there remains just one narrow lane for travel into the city. A long, slow traffic jam is now the rule rather than the exception. Supplies are not getting into the city fast enough or in great enough quantity to keep the city's population thriving. The city is literally being choked off from the outside world because of a trash-littered freeway.

Take this scenario and imagine it's in your arteries that feed blood to your heart, a working muscle that needs oxygen and nutrients like any other part of your body. Your first warning sign of a traffic jam (constricted blood flow) is gripping chest pain called *angina pectoris*. Or worse yet, a clogged heart artery completely blocks blood flow and you suffer a full-blown heart attack. If garbage along the highway to your brain blocks or slows the supplies it needs (primarily oxygen), a stroke occurs leaving those portions of your brain starved and damaged. Elsewhere in your body, arteries supplying your legs or arms may also become blocked, killing off precious tissue by starving it from much needed oxygen and nutrients.

The heart people call this process *atherosclerosis*—a buildup of garbage or debris called *plaque* made up of a cholesterol-fat mixture and other gunk. Plaque in the arteries that feed your heart leads to heart disease and eventually to a heart attack. Elsewhere, such as in your brain, plaque buildup causes stroke—a brain attack. Just like debris that accumulates on a roadside, plaque buildup doesn't happen overnight. The process takes many years, actually a lifetime to develop. Why cholesterol, fat, and other unmentionables end up as debris that eventually may clog your arteries is another traffic story.

## The Real Scoop on Cholesterol

Knowing that cholesterol is to blame for traffic jams in your arteries gives you the impression that if you can avoid the stuff, you'll be heart attack free. Not so. Cholesterol is good. Hard to believe, but this fatty wax-like substance is absolutely crucial for your body to function. For starters, your sex hormones are made from cholesterol; no cholesterol, no sex. But, cholesterol can become problematic when too much circulates around the highways of your body and the vehicles responsible for cholesterol's transportation drive out of control.

Cholesterol is made daily right in your body and shipped out from the liver into the bloodstream for transport from head to toe. You also get cholesterol from your daily fare. Any food that comes from an animal contains cholesterol (like humans, animals make cholesterol for the same uses). Milk, any type of meat, fish, and eggs contain cholesterol, but only milligram amounts, which is far less than the amount of protein or fat in these foods.

How cholesterol makes its way through the body is central to the heart-disease-and-traffic-jam story. Like other fats, cholesterol is not soluble in water and is unable to travel alone through water-based blood. It would be like mixing oil with water—can't do it! As a result, cholesterol and other fats must get a ride as passengers in a special "bus" called a *lipoprotein;* it's fatty on the inside for its passengers and watery on the outside to mix with blood. As passengers inside the bus, cholesterol and fat travel freely through the body. In fact, some lipoprotein buses stop at preassigned "bus stops" where the doors open and cholesterol passengers hop off where needed. Fat, which is often called *triglyceride,* is also dropped off where needed such as in muscle and fat tissue for storage.

Several types of buses are responsible for transporting cholesterol. Two important ones are: *LDL* or *Low-Density Lipoprotein,* the primary bus responsible for delivering cholesterol throughout the body; and *HDL* or *High-Density Lipoprotein,* a clean-up bus that picks up wandering cholesterol along your roadways (arteries) and elsewhere, bringing it back to bus headquarters (the liver) for eventual removal from the body. HDL is often dubbed the "good" cholesterol because of its clean-up role. The cholesterol in these different lipoproteins is the same, but as you will see, it's the low-density lipoprotein bus carrying the cholesterol that can be troublesome.

### *Your Arteries—The LDL-HDL Story*

When the bus system runs smoothly, roadways stay open, free from congested traffic. But problems may arise with the LDL bus. If the bus driver becomes mad or irritated (in your system this is called *LDL oxidation*), the bus drives recklessly and the cholesterol passengers are thrown from the bus, strewn along artery walls rather than in needy tissues where they belong. When oxidized or irritated, the LDL bus rams into the roadside—your artery walls, where the cholesterol passengers are dumped. The LDL bus is more likely to crash along roadsides that are "sticky" or bumpy. Also, too many LDL buses (high levels) cause traffic congestion in your arteries and as a result, more cholesterol gets dumped at the side of the road. It's no surprise then why LDLs are often referred to as the "bad" cholesterol, or more accurately, the "bad carrier" of cholesterol.

Years of oxidized LDLs ramming into artery walls leaves your roadways narrow and clogged, paving the way for a heart attack or stroke. Several factors lead to the destruction caused by oxidized LDL buses. Smoking, for example, is known to make LDL bus drivers go crazy. Another culprit is a poor intake of certain vitamins such as vitamins C and E as well as other nutrients that prevent the LDLs from becoming irritated. High levels of circulating homocysteine (an amino acid made in your body from protein) is thought to injure artery walls, making them more prone to an LDL bus ramming into the damaged site and causing even further injury. (If heart disease runs in your family, see your physician about getting homocysteine levels checked.)

Besides LDL buses running amuck, too few HDLs also spells trouble for heart health. Since HDLs help clean up loose cholesterol, too few of these buses in circulation boost chances for clogged roadways and heart disease. Not enough HDL roaming around your blood vessels is similar to too few public works vehicles assigned to keep roadways free of debris. There are a number of reasons, including diet, that make HDL levels go up or down. Regular exercise, for example, helps boost levels of HDLs, explaining in part why exercisers have a lower risk for heart disease. Also, women (before the age of menopause) have higher HDL levels than men, giving them some extra protection. This helps explain why their heart disease risk is lower than men's during their premenopausal years.

Since LDL and HDL both play a part in the process of heart disease, one bad and the other good, it's not surprising that the level of these buses helps predict heart-disease risk. High circulating levels of LDL are dangerous for your heart. And the *lower* the level of HDL, the higher your risk. Also, a measure of total cholesterol in circulation which represents cholesterol held by LDLs, HDLs, and other types of lipoprotein buses also helps predict risk. In general, the higher your cholesterol, the greater your risk of a heart attack. A measure of circulating fat, called *triglyceride,* also helps rank your risk for heart disease.

Getting your blood cholesterol level checked is a must when it comes to tracking your heart health. See your physician for this simple test, which requires a sample of blood. Sometimes health fairs held at shopping malls or local pharmacy stores offer cholesterol testing for free or for a nominal charge. A great idea, but it's best to see your physician for a complete test. Ideally, you should have what's called a *lipoprotein screen,* which means LDL and HDL as well as total cholesterol levels are measured. Armed with this information you can assess your risk. Check the "Cholesterol Countdown" chart for heart-healthy numbers.

The Simple Six Eating Plan described in this book is designed to help you lower total cholesterol and LDL cholesterol levels as well as raise HDL cholesterol. As you will see, many of the 101 Miracle Foods protect your heart by lowering cholesterol levels or by keeping LDLs from becoming oxidized and damaging artery walls.

### How Your Body Feels About High Blood Pressure

If clogged arteries from cholesterol buildup are similar to a roadway jammed with debris, then high blood pressure is analogous to rigid roadways that don't expand to accommodate the flow of traffic. For 50 million Americans, high blood pressure, called *hypertension,* puts a strain on the heart and boosts the chances of suffering from a heart attack or stroke. In fact, according to a recent survey, more than 700,000 strokes occur every year, 40 percent more than previous estimates. Stroke can strike anyone at any time, as it did my friend, Randal. Ironically, he came to see me about his high blood pressure just days before his massive stroke. He's recovering but, needless to say, he is keeping watch over his blood pressure readings.

Blood pressure is simply the amount of force generated by blood against the artery walls. If you have ever had your blood

### Cholesterol Countdown*

*How do your numbers compare? (Note: Cholesterol and lipoprotein screens measure cholesterol in milligrams per 1 deciliter of blood, or mg/dL.)*

| Cholesterol Level (mg/dL) | Desirable | Borderline | High-Risk |
|---|---|---|---|
| Total cholesterol | less than 200 | 200–239 | 240 or higher |
| LDL | less than 130 | 130–159 | 160 or higher |
| HDL | 35 or higher | less than 35 | less than 35 |

\* Figures from the U.S. Department of Health and Human Services

Cholesterol tests may often include a measure of triglycerides (fat). Readings below 200 mg/dL are desirable.

pressure taken, you know it's expressed in two numbers such as 120/80 mm Hg (read: 120 over 80), and the units are a measure of force. When your heart, which is a pump, contracts or beats, the force exerted is the first or higher number called the *systolic blood pressure*. Between beats or during relaxation of the heart, the blood pressure is lower. This lower number is called the *diastolic blood pressure*. Throughout the day, your blood pressure changes depending on your activities: When you are resting, for example, your blood pressure reading should be lower than when you are exercising or doing yard work.

A blood pressure of 120/80 is considered normal. Below this number is also healthy but a reading below 90/60 needs some looking into by your physician. The more likely problem is a blood pressure that is too high. Up to 139/89 is considered okay, with 140/90 defined as hypertensive. The higher numbers indicate the blood vessel walls are more rigid and the blood then must exert a greater force as it moves through the system. This puts a strain on the heart as well as the blood vessels and arteries, leading to greater chances for developing heart disease and stroke.

Besides wreaking havoc on your heart health, high blood pressure goes unnoticed unless you are looking for it. You cannot feel high blood pressure. Often called the "silent killer," hypertension can go undetected for years, causing long-term damage and finally showing itself when it may be too late. Since one in four Americans have high blood pressure, get it checked.

Using an inflatable arm cuff, this painless test can be done in a matter of minutes. Many pharmacies often have free testing stations. Also see your physician for testing. Know that blood pressure varies throughout the day, so one reading isn't enough to determine your blood pressure health. If several readings taken over several days fall into the hypertension range then you have high blood pressure.

Treating high blood pressure is crucial since your risk for a heart attack and stroke is now much greater. Options include medication prescribed by your physician, weight loss, and changes in your current diet. If you are on blood pressure medication, it is crucial you stay on it. If you are trying to lower your blood pressure with changes in your diet, you must confer with your physician for advice. But don't stop taking your medication without clearance from your doc.

One of the most effective ways to help control blood pressure, not only to lower your existing reading but to prevent further increases, is weight loss. Carrying around extra fat weight puts a strain on the heart and contributes to boosting blood pressure. Also, regular exercise helps improve blood pressure control.

Exciting new research over the past few years has shown that eating certain foods on a regular basis can be as effective in lowering blood pressure as taking medications. Eating a diet that is loaded with plenty of fruits and vegetables—about 8 to 10 servings daily, has a powerful impact on lower blood pressure readings. My Simple Six Eating Plan ensures that you get the right amount of fruits and vegetables to lower your blood pressure.

Other research shows that eating foods rich in fiber may also lower blood pressure. Certain foods that supply calcium, magnesium, and potassium may also put a dent in hypertension. And while for years well-wishers have put down their saltshakers in hopes of controlling hypertension, researchers now feel that sodium is not the huge threat it was once thought to be.

## How You Can Eat Away Heart Disease and High Blood Pressure

Your heart health is in your control. While some of the factors that boost your heart-disease risk may be untouchable, such as your family history (unfortunately, we can't pick our parents), virtually all others rest in your hands—whether you choose not to smoke or to get regular exercise, for example. But my intention with this book is not to burden you with every lifestyle option that can boost heart health. Instead, I focus on your most potent and powerful ally—food. One hundred and one foods, to be exact. Many of these foods, when put to the test in well-controlled research studies, help boost heart health and lower high blood pressure.

### *Diet Basics for a Healthy Heart*

My Simple Six Eating Plan is all about *simple.* I assure you that after seeing the basics in Chapter Two, you will find that the Simple Six is an eating scheme you can do easily, without tedious planning, special foods, or weighing portions. I know from experience that few people have the time or the intense motivation needed to follow very low-fat or strict vegetarian eating programs. I prefer to set up a plan with foods people enjoy. And as you will read, even chocolate, eggs, and butter can fit in your Simple Six Eating Plan.

# *Your Personal Eating Plan*

There are so many things to think about when choosing "good" foods. You need to separate the heart-friendly monounsaturated fats from the heart-stopping saturated fats. Then of course there's the need to increase the amount of the good HDL cholesterol and reduce the level of the artery-clogging LDL cholesterol. And we all know that fiber is good but sugar is bad (sometimes). And animal protein is good but plant protein is better. Antioxidants, of course, should be on your plate, along with the B vitamins and minerals like potassium, calcium, and magnesium. And don't forget those phytochemicals that fight off heart disease.

Because there are so many substances in food that work together to keep the heart healthy, the task of getting them all on your plate on a regular basis can be overwhelming. That's why I have created an eating plan for you that is straightforward, easy to follow, and, well, downright *simple*. I call it the Simple Six Eating Plan. This eating program is designed with your needs in mind: You have limited time for planning, shopping, and cooking meals; you are interested in eating foods for a healthy heart but not keen on turning your life around to follow an exotic, complicated program, and you want an eating plan that's easy to follow so you can make it part of your lifestyle. Sounds like you? Then the Simple Six Eating Plan *is* for you.

## The Simple Six Eating Plan

The "six" reflects the six different groups or types of foods that make up your eating program. This includes a wide array of nutrients and substances in foods that make for a healthy heart. These different food categories supply your body and heart with those nutrients and substances. There are some 50-plus nutrients, along with phytochemicals needed for good health as well as for fending off heart disease and high blood pressure. Working with six categories of foods makes eating simple and takes any confusion out of setting up an eating plan that meets your personal needs.

First, let's meet each of the six food categories—an overview of heart-healthy ingredients in each group, a guide to serving sizes in each category, and a listing of foods for each group. Notice that each of the six groups is identified with a simple food symbol.

Next, let's take a look at your personal plan. I designed an easy-to-follow guide identifying the number of food servings in each category to eat daily based on your needs. The same food-group symbols are used to help you visually track your daily meal plan. Find these same food group symbols in Part Two of this book when selecting any of the 101 Miracle Foods. These symbols will help you identify how these foods fit in with your eating plan.

*Meet the "Simple Six"*

### 1. Soy (soybeans and other soy foods) and Other Beans (legumes)

Central to the Simple Six Eating Plan is two daily servings of soy to supply heart-healthy soy protein and soy phytochemicals called isoflavones. Soy foods and other beans also supply you with a great source of soluble fiber, the type that helps lower blood cholesterol. Along with protein and fiber, these beans come with an array of vitamins and minerals, and some soy foods are a good source of calcium as well as heart-healthy monounsaturated fat with no cholesterol.

## Soy and Other Beans

One serving contains approximately 50–100 calories and 7–13 grams of protein. (Serving size varies.)*

| *Soybean and Soy Food:* | *Beans or Legumes (cooked):* |
| --- | --- |
| Tofu, firm, 4 ounces | Black beans, 1/2 cup |
| Baked tofu, 2 ounces | Chickpeas, 1/2 cup |
| Miso, 1/4 cup | Navy beans, 1/2 cup |
| Natto, 1/4 cup | Refried beans,*** 1/2 cup |
| Tempeh, 1/4 cup | White beans, 1/2 cup |
| Soymilk, 1 cup | Peas, split, 1/2 cup |

Soyburger, 1 pattie

Soy "ground beef," 2 ounces

Soy hot dog, 1 weiner

Soy sandwich "meat" slices, 2 ounces

Soy breakfast links, 2

Soy breakfast patty, 1

Soy flour, defatted, 1/4 cup

Soybeans, cooked, 1/2 cup

Soynuts, 1/8 cup

Isolated soy protein powder,** Health Source® brand, 1/2 ounce

Isolated soy protein powder, flavored, Health Source® brand, 1 ounce

Textured vegetable protein, made with water, 1/4 cup

* One serving, in some cases, may not match serving size indicated on food packages or in other sections of this book. Serving sizes were adjusted to accommodate differences in calorie and protein content of various soy foods.

** A serving per manufacturer's label is 1 ounce (premeasured scoop in canister).

*** Check label for added fat. Select fat-free versions to avoid addition of hydrogenated fats.

## 2. Grains—pasta, rice, whole grains such as barley, breads, cereals, potatoes, winter squashes, corn, and crackers

This group takes up some space on your plate. All of the grain foods supply a wealth of carbohydrates, fiber, B vitamins (particularly folic acid), vitamins A and E in some foods, minerals such as magnesium and calcium, and phytochemicals. Processed grain products such as crackers, chips, or plain (white) pasta and bread are generally lower in fiber and other nutrients. They also have added salt. Check the label, as some of these foods may have added fat, oftentimes the unfriendly hydrogenated fats. These foods should be selected less frequently.

## Grains

One serving contains approximately 80 calories. (Size varies depending on food item.)

| | |
|---|---|
| Bagel, 1/2 | Popcorn, air popped, 3 cups |
| Bran, wheat, 1/2 cup | Rice, brown, 1/3 cup |
| Bread, whole grain | Corn, cooked, 1/2 cup |
|    (wheat, barley, rye), 1 slice | Potato, baked with skin, 1 small |
| Cereal, ready-to-eat, | Squash, butternut, acorn, 1 cup |
|    whole grain, 1/2–3/4 cup | Pumpkin, cooked, 1 cup |
| Cereal, cooked (oatmeal, | Wheat germ, 3 tbsp. |
|    whole corn grits), 1/2 cup | Rice cakes, whole grain, 2 |
| English muffin, whole grain, 1/2 | Tortilla, whole corn or flour, 1 |
| Pasta, whole grain, 1/2 cup | |
| Pita bread, whole grain, 1/2 | |

| *Use Less Frequently:* | *Use Sparingly:* |
|---|---|
| Breads and rolls, white, 1 slice | Muffin, bakery type, 1 small |
| Crackers, snack type, 8 | Chips, 1 ounce |
| Granola low-fat cereal, 1/4 | Cake, no icing, 2-inch square |
| Pancake, 1 | Brownie, 1 1/2-inch square |
| Muffin, low-fat, 1 small | |
| Cookies, low-fat or fat-free, 2 small | |
| Waffle, 1 (4 inches wide) | |

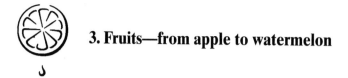

# 3. Fruits—from apple to watermelon

Fruits supply plenty of carbohydrate energy and fiber. They also deliver a wide array of vitamins, notably vitamin C, carotenes, minerals, especially potassium and a staggering number of phytochemicals to keep you healthy.

## Fruits

One serving contains approximately 60 calories. (See list for fruit and fruit juice serving size.)

Apple, 1 small

Apricots, 4 fresh (or 8 halves dried)

Blackberries, blueberries, etc., 3/4 cup

Cantaloupe, 1 cup cubed

Cherries, 12 fresh

Dates, 3

Figs, 2

Grapefruit, 1/2

Grapes, 15

Guava, 1/2 med.

Fruit juice, 1/2 cup
   apple, orange

Fruit juice, 1/3 cup
   cranberry, prune

Kiwifruit, 1 med.

Mango, 1 small

Nectarine, 1 small

Orange, 1 small

Papaya, 1 cup cubed

Peach, 1 med.

Pear, 1 small

Pineapple, 3/4 cup cubed

Plums, 2 small

Strawberries, 1 1/4 cups

Tangerines, 2 small

Watermelon, 1 1/4 cup cubed

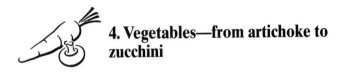

## 4. Vegetables—from artichoke to zucchini

The produce section, as well as the frozen food aisle, is full of many different vegetables. These wonders of Mother Nature supply plenty of fiber, vitamins (A, C, and B vitamins), minerals, and a slew of healing phytochemicals.

## Vegetables

One serving contains approximately 25 calories. (See list for serving sizes.)

Artichoke, 1 med.

Asparagus, 1/2 cup cooked

Beans, green, 1/2 cup cooked

Beets, 1/2 cup

Broccoli, 1/2 cup cooked
　or 1 cup raw

Brussels sprouts, 1/2 cup cooked

Cabbage, 1 cup raw shredded
　or 1/2 cup cooked

Carrot, 1 cup raw sliced
　or 1/2 cup cooked

Cauliflower, 1 cup raw
　or 1/2 cup cooked

Celery, 1 cup raw slices

Cucumber, 1 cup slices

Eggplant, 1/2 cup cooked

Green, 1 cup raw or 1/2 cup cooked

Mushrooms, 1 cup raw sliced

Okra, 1/2 cooked

Onion, 1/2 cup cooked

Peppers, 1 med.

Radishes, 10 raw

Rutabaga, 1/2 cup cooked

Spinach, 1 cup raw, or
　1/2 cup cooked

Sprouts, bean, 1 cup

Squash, summer, 3/4 cup cooked

Tomato, 1 med.

Tomato juice, 1/2 cup

Turnips, 1/2 cup cooked

Vegetable juice, 1/2 cup

Zucchini, 3/4 cup cooked

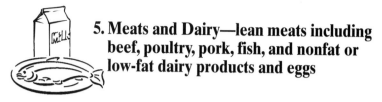

## 5. Meats and Dairy—lean meats including beef, poultry, pork, fish, and nonfat or low-fat dairy products and eggs

These foods supply an excellent source of protein. Meats provide a variety of vitamins and minerals, especially iron and zinc. Dairy products are a major source of calcium. Always select lean or extra lean cuts of meats, remove skin from poultry, and use cooking methods such as broiling, grilling, and microwaving that don't use added fats. Select dairy products that are fat-free or reduced fat versions. Use full fat varieties sparingly.

## Meats and Dairy

One serving contains approximately 80 to 110 calories and 8 to 20 grams of protein. (See list for serving sizes.)

*Meats*

Beef,* lean cuts, 3 ounces cooked
Fish, fresh or frozen, 3 ounces cooked
Fish, canned
   Salmon, 3 ounces
   Sardines, 4 med.
   Tuna, in water, 3 ounces
Pork,* lean cuts, 3 ounces
Poultry,* no skin
   Chicken, turkey, 3 ounces cooked
   Ground poultry, 3 ounces cooked
Processed meat,*
   low-fat or fat-free, 3 ounces
Shellfish
   Clams, 15 med.
   Crab, lobster, 3 ounces cooked
   Oysters, 12 med.
   Shrimp, 15 med.

*Dairy*

Cheese*
   Low-fat or fat-free, 3 ounces
   Parmesan, grated, 1/4 cup
   Low-fat or fat-free cottage
     cheese, 3/4 cup
   Low-fat or fat-free ricotta,
     3/4 cup
Milk, fat-free, 1/2%, 1%, 1 cup
Yogurt, fat-free, low-fat, 1 cup
Eggs
   Egg, whole, 1 1/2 large
   Egg whites, 4
   Egg substitute, 3/4 cup

*Use less frequently:*
Ice cream,* nonfat, 1/2 cup
Frozen yogurt,* nonfat, 1/2 cup

---

* These items vary in fat content. Select those with lowest saturated fat content; see specific food items in Part Two.

# 6. Fats—oils, avocado, nuts, and seeds

While high in calories, these foods supply heart-friendly fats and essential fats along with vitamin E crucial for good health. Some of these foods, such as nuts, also contain disease-fighting phytochemicals. In an effort to control calorie intake, especially if weight loss is desired, pay close attention to serving sizes and the use of added fats in prepared dishes. Check the label on margarine products and salad dressings for hydrogenated fat content. Keep hydrogenated fats to a minimum.

## Fats

One serving contains approximately 45 calories. (See list, as serving size varies.)

Avocado, 1/8 med.

Butter,* 1 tsp.

Mayonnaise, reduced-fat, 1 tbsp.
  regular, 1 tsp.

Margarine,* reduced-fat, 1 tbsp.
  regular, 1 tsp.

Nuts, unsalted
  almonds, 6
  Brazil, 2
  cashews, 6
  peanuts, 10
  pecans, whole, 2
  walnuts, 2 whole or 4 halves

Nut butters, 1 tbsp.
  peanut butter
  almond butter

Oils
  canola, 1 tsp.
  olive, 1 tsp.
  peanut, 1 tsp.
  corn, 1 tsp.
  safflower, 1 tsp.
  sunflower, 1 tsp.

Seeds
  flax, 1 tbsp.
  pumpkin, 1 tbsp.
  sesame, 1 tbsp.
  sunflower, 1 tbsp.

Salad dressings*
  reduced-fat, 2 tbsp.
  fat-free, 3 tbsp.
  regular, 1 tbsp.

* Contains saturated or hydrogenated fats, use less frequently than items rich in monounsaturated fats. See specific items in Part Two for more information.

### Serving Sense

Did you pour a half-cup of cereal in the bowl or was it more like a cup? A tablespoon or teaspoon of dressing over your salad? When it gets right down to it, most of us "eyeball" our portions. The problem is, most of the time we underestimate how much we are serving ourselves. And the problem with that is the extra calories that may lead to weight gain. To avoid "super-sized" servings, I suggest you purchase a set of plastic measuring cups including teaspoon and tablespoon measures. And then, before eating, measure each food item. Do this for a few days to get a feel for what an accurate serving size, a half-cup serving of cooked pasta, for example, looks like on your plate.

Another way to keep track of serving sizes is to use familiar items as size equivalents. Here's what I mean:

- 3-ounce serving of cooked fish, beef, or poultry = the size of a deck of cards
- 1-ounce serving of reduced-fat cheese = the size of a set of dice or a 1-inch cube
- 1 medium apple or other fruit = the size of a tennis ball
- 1 tablespoon of peanut butter or dressing = size of half a ping-pong ball
- 1 teaspoon of oil = the size of the tip of your thumb

## Your Personal Simple Six Eating Plan

Depending upon your calorie needs, there is a Simple Six Eating Plan for you. The number of servings from each of the Simple Six groups are indicated for each calorie level. To determine how many calories you need for your current weight simply use the "Caloric Needs Formula" as a guide:

## Caloric Needs Formula

If your age is 30 to 49, then multiply your current weight by:

> 12 for women and 13 for men.
>
> *Example:* A 48-year-old woman weighing 150 lb.
>> 150 lb. x 12 = 1800 calories needed per day

If your age is 50 or over, then multiply your current weight by:

> 11 for women and 12 for men.
>
> *Example:* A 55-year-old man weighing 170 lb.
>> 170 lb. x 12 = 2040 calories needed per day

This formula, multiplying your weight by a factor, approximates how many calories you need daily. Many factors can change this, such as activity level. With regular exercise, such as walking three miles daily or attending aerobics or other fitness classes, your calorie needs can go up substantially. So use this equation as a starting point. Your best bet is to track the food you eat over several days and calculate how many calories you average daily.

## Simple Six Guide

| Daily Calories | Soy* & Beans | Grains | Fruits | Vegetables | Meat** & Dairy | Fat |
|---|---|---|---|---|---|---|
| 1200 | 3 | 4 | 4 | 4 | 2 | 3 |
| 1400 | 3 | 5 | 5 | 5 | 2 | 3 |
| 1600 | 3 | 6 | 5 | 5 | 3 | 4 |
| 1800 | 3 | 7 | 5 | 5 | 4 | 5 |
| 2000 | 3 1/2 | 8 | 5 | 5 | 4 | 6 |
| 2200 | 4 | 9 | 5 | 6 | 4 | 7 |
| 2400 | 4 | 10 | 6 | 6 | 4 | 8 |

\* At least two soy servings daily

\** At least two dairy servings daily

This reflects your personal calorie needs. If weight loss is desired, then increase the number of calories you burn through exercise, and decrease the number of calories you consume. (More on this in the next section.) Find your calorie level in the Simple Six Guide at left and see how many servings from each of the six food categories you need to keep your heart healthy.

## Simple Six Menu Plans

To give you an idea of how a Simple Six plan "looks," check out these menus. The nutritional profile for each is listed.

### Menu #1: 2300 calories

**BREAKFAST:**

1 cup hot 9-grain cereal made with 1 oz. (one scoop) of isolated soy powder topped with 1 cup sliced strawberries

1 cup nonfat vanilla yogurt

1 slice whole-grain bread, toasted

1 banana

hot tea (green or black) with lemon

**LUNCH:**

Pita tuna sandwich:

tuna salad made with fresh chopped coriander, red onion, and 1/2 cup garbanzo beans

plus 1 tbsp. reduced-fat mayonnaise

1 cup All Red Salad (see page 80 for recipe)

1 cup fruit salad (melon and blueberries)

**SNACK:**

1 med. orange

2 stalks celery

1/8 cup soynuts

**DINNER:**

1 baked potato topped with 1/2 cup canned sloppy Joe mixed with 1/2 cup black beans

1 cup steamed cauliflower with 1 oz. grated Parmesan cheese

1 cup mixed green salad with 1 tbsp. olive oil vinaigrette

Oaty Apple Crisp (see page 193 for recipe)

**Nutritional Profile: Total Calories 2300 with 2 1/2 servings of soy**

Protein: 114 grams   Fat: 60 grams   Carbohydrate: 325 grams   Fiber: 44 grams

(or)

| **Nutrition Facts** | |
| --- | --- |
| Serving Size 1 Day's menu | |
| Amount per Serving | |
| Calories 2300    540 Calories from fat | |
| | % Daily Value |
| Total Fat 60g | 92% |
| Saturated Fat 14g | 70% |
| Cholesterol 52mg | 17% |
| Sodium 2200mg | 96% |
| Total Carbohydrate 325g | 108% |
| Dietary Fiber 44g | 177% |
| Protein 114g | |
| Vitamin A 130% • Vitamin C 732% | |
| Calcium 146% • Iron 113% | |
| Folic Acid 153% • Vitamin E 400% | |

*Menu #2: 1800 Calories*

**BRUNCH:**

2 "egg" omelet made with egg substitute filled with 1/2 cup cooked spinach, mushrooms, and 1 oz. goat cheese

2 breakfast links (made with soy—Morningstar Farms brand)

2 flax seed muffins topped with 1 tbsp. jam

1 cup melon and berries

6 oz. orange juice

tea with lemon

**SNACK:**

4 whole-grain crackers spread with 1 tbsp. soybutter

1 nectarine

1/2 cup cucumber slices dipped with 1/4 cup plain yogurt blended with herbs

**DINNER:**

Tomatoes Stuffed with Tofu (see page 278 for recipe)

1 cup Rice-Lentil Salad (see page 233 for recipe)

1 cup spinach tossed with 1/2 cup garbanzo beans and 1 tbsp. vinaigrette dressing

1 cup sliced strawberries over small whole-grain waffle drizzled with honey

**Nutritional Profile: Total Calories 1800 with 2 1/2 servings of soy**

Protein: 96 grams   Fat: 60 grams   Carbohydrate: 250 grams   Fiber: 40 grams

(or)

| **Nutrition Facts** | |
| :--- | ---: |
| Serving Size 1 Day's menu | |
| **Amount per Serving** | |
| Calories 1800    540 Calories from fat | |
| | % Daily Value |
| Total Fat 60g | 93% |
| Saturated Fat 14g | 70% |
| Cholesterol 116mg | 39% |
| Sodium 2270mg | 95% |
| Total Carbohydrate 250g | 85% |
| Dietary Fiber 40g | 160% |
| Protein 96g | |
| Vitamin A 320% • Vitamin C 525% | |
| Calcium 100%   •   Iron 150% | |
| Folic Acid 150% • Vitamin E 170% | |

## *Menu #3: 1200 Calories*

### BREAKFAST:
Tropical Blender Blast smoothie (see page 287 for recipe)

1/2 toasted whole-wheat bagel topped with 1 tbsp. jam

### LUNCH:
Veggie burger:
  1 patty
  1 whole-grain bun
  tomato and onion slices

1 cup coleslaw made with fat-free dressing (1 1/2 tbsp.)

8 oz. skim milk

### SNACK:
iced tea with lemon

### DINNER:
3 oz. grilled halibut topped with dill-lemon sauce

1 cup green beans with crushed garlic

1/2 cup wild rice pilaf

1 cup arugala and endive salad dressed with 2 tsp. olive oil-vinegar dressing

1/2 cup fresh berries topped with a dollop of vanilla yogurt

**Nutritional Profile: Total Calories 1200 with 2 servings of soy**

Protein: 73 grams   Fat: 18 grams   Carbohydrate: 200 grams   Fiber: 28 grams

(or)

| **Nutrition Facts** Serving Size 1 Day's menu | |
|---|---|
| Amount per Serving | |
| Calories 1200    162 Calories from fat | |
| | % Daily Value |
| Total Fat 18g | 28% |
|    Saturated Fat 4g | 21% |
| Cholesterol 42mg | 14% |
| Sodium 1400mg | 59% |
| Total Carbohydrate 200g | 67% |
|    Dietary Fiber 28g | 110% |
| Protein 73g | |
| Vitamin A 76%  •  Vitamin C 340% Calcium 80%  •  Iron 70% Folic Acid 105%  •  Vitamin E 200% | |

## Weighty Matters: Using the Simple Six Eating Plan for Weight Loss

Put bluntly, extra pounds strain your heart. Being overweight increases the chances of developing heart disease and hypertension, and boosts the likelihood of suffering from a heart attack or stroke. According to statistics, about a third of all adult Americans are at risk due to creeping obesity. But the good news is that losing weight, as little as five to ten pounds, can work wonders for your heart. Losing excess weight may:

- lower levels of the cholesterol bad-guy, LDLs.
- boost levels of the cholesterol good-guy, HDLs.
- reduce unhealthy blood pressure.
- lower blood fat levels called triglycerides.
- improve blood sugar control in diabetics and prediabetics.

The decision to lose weight should be based on health reasons rather than on a personal decision to "look better" or "please a spouse." Losing weight and keeping it off is no small task. As you may well know, few people succeed in losing and keeping excess weight off for at least a year. While the reasons for weight-loss failure are many, most experts agree that dieters oftentimes fail to make *committed lifestyle changes* that they intend to keep, such as regular physical activity and eating a diet lower in fat and higher in fruits, vegetables, and whole grains.

Your decision to lose weight should include the advice of a physician who can assess your current risk factors for heart disease and stroke, matched with your weight. For starters, check the "Tipping the Scales" chart which shows the recently revised numbers from the National Institute of Health that serve as cutoffs points for "overweight" and "obese." The government and many health professionals use the BMI (Body Mass Index), a measure of weight relative to height, as an indicator of excess weight. The BMI equals a person's weight measured in kilograms divided by height measured in meters and then squared. Instead of giving you the task of figuring out your own BMI, simply refer to the chart and find your height. Then check out what weight puts you in "overweight" or "obese" categories.

According to government standards, a BMI of 25 is defined as "overweight." As an example, a person 5'8" who weighs 164 has a BMI over 25 and is defined as overweight (see chart on the next page). If that same person weighed 197 pounds or more, they would have a BMI of 30 or over and be defined as "obese." An obese person should seek the advice of a physician and lose weight to improve health. The goal is to lose about one to two pounds a week until about 10 percent of an individual's body weight is lost, 20 pounds for a 200-pound person, for example. This amount of weight loss will improve heart health significantly.

For some individuals, further weight loss may be necessary but should involve a physician's advice that weight loss is medically necessary. For example, Bob came to me for diet help when his physician advised weight loss. His blood pressure was high, as were his cholesterol levels. Bob was 35 pounds over-

## Tipping the Scales?

Use this chart to determine where your weight "falls." Look for your height in the left-hand column and then move across to determine if your BMI* lies below the "overweight" cutoff (BMI = 25) or exceeds this and is closer to the "obese" BMI of 30.

**Example:** A woman who is 5'6" weighing 165 lb. is defined as overweight. A woman of the same height weighing 187 lb. is defined as obese.

| | Overweight and Obese Cutoff Points | |
|---|---|---|
| **Height (inches)** | **BMI = 25 Overweight (pounds)** | **BMI = 30 Obese (pounds)** |
| 58 | 119 | 147 |
| 60 | 128 | 153 |
| 62 | 136 | 164 |
| 64 | 145 | 174 |
| 66 | 155 | 186 |
| 68 | 164 | 197 |
| 70 | 174 | 207 |
| 72 | 185 | 221 |
| 74 | 194 | 233 |
| 76 | 205 | 246 |

* BMI = Body Mass Index, a measure of body weight relative to height. BMI is equal to weight (kilograms) divided by height (meters)$^2$.

weight and ended up losing 20 of those in about 5 months with the help of a walking program and some calorie cutting. His doc was more than pleased since his blood pressure and cholesterol readings both fell into the healthy range, all without medication. As a result, further weight loss was not stressed by Bob's physician. He does keep up with his walking program to control any further weight gain.

If you are "overweight" (a BMI of 25 but less than 30) you should resist further weight gain, and definitely lose weight if you have two or more weight-related risk factors: high blood pressure, high blood cholesterol, diabetes, impaired ability to tolerate glucose (prediabetic condition), or if your waist measurement exceeds 35 inches if you are a woman or 40 inches if you are a man. Carrying excess fat around your waist or in the abdominal region is dangerous to your heart's health and boosts your risk for a heart attack, high blood pressure, diabetes, and other conditions. Your physician can help you determine whether you have any of these weight-related health risks.

### Rx for Weight Loss with the Simple Six

Losing weight is simple: Take in fewer calories than you burn. The tough part is making that happen. When you set your mind to losing weight, you must commit yourself to making lifestyle changes that lead to a weight loss that you can maintain. Losing and regaining weight is not the cycle you want to be on, as research clearly shows on-again-off-again weight loss causes its own set of health problems. Losing weight and keeping it off means including regular activity as well as eating a low-fat diet packed with fruits, vegetables, and whole grains.

Losing weight means eating less and being more active. A recommended rate of weight loss is one to two pounds per week. To meet this goal, you must create a calorie deficit of 500 to 1000 calories daily. In other words, you must eat less and exercise more. That amounts to a 500 to 1000 calorie loss for the day, and by the end of the week this translates to a one- to two-pound fat loss.

Most of the 500 to 1000 calorie daily loss should come from eating less by cutting back on portion sizes and foods such as sugary or fatty treats that merely add "empty" calories to your diet rather than health-boosting nutrients. Another 100 to 300 calories should come from being more active. About 45 minutes of moderately intense walking at least five days a week is recommended (see your physician first before your start an exercise program).

The Simple Six Eating Plan makes a perfect match for your effort to lose weight. The Simple Six is designed to be low in fat; about 20 percent to less than 30 percent of the calories are from fat (most of which are the heart-healthy fats). With the Simple Six you are eating a minimum of eight servings of fruits and vegetables daily, which ensures plenty of filling fiber to help lessen feelings of hunger while keeping your intestinal tract healthy. Besides fiber, you'll meet your need for various vitamins and minerals crucial in fat burning.

It's simple to get started using the Simple Six for weight loss. Using the Simple Six Guide on page 22, find your current calorie needs based on the formula I gave you on the same page, or use an estimate of your own from previous record keeping of what you typically eat each day. Now, take yourself down two levels, or 400 calories. This calorie cutting, along with your increased activity, will help you reach a minimum of a 500-calorie loss per day, or about one pound of fat loss per week.

Let's use my friend Dave as an example. He is 51 years old, weighs 200 pounds, and is 6 feet tall. Using the BMI chart on page 29, Dave is overweight, and because he also has high blood cholesterol and hypertension, his physician has advised him to begin a walking program and to lose weight. Using my formula, he needs 2400 calories daily to maintain his current weight. But to lose weight he should take his calorie intake down to 2000 calories and follow the serving allotments for each category from the Simple Six Guide.

Dave was amazed when I set up this menu plan for him. He was in disbelief that he could lose weight while eating "all that food." Many people, like my friend Dave, are used to eating foods rich in calories from added fat and not accustomed to fresh fruits and vegetables. And becoming familiar with true serving sizes was also an eye-opening experience for Dave and many other people I work with on weight loss. We have come to expect "super-sized" servings at restaurants and elsewhere. Dave had no idea that one serving of pasta was just a half cup. But with the plentiful servings of fruits and vegetables, Dave walked away feeling full.

### *Dave's 2000 Calorie Simple Six Weight Loss Meal Plan:*

#### BREAKFAST:
1 cup ready-to-eat oat cereal

topped with one banana sliced and

1 cup of soymilk (low-fat)

1/2 bagel, toasted, spread with 1 tbsp. berry jam

#### MORNING SNACK:
1/2 cup Power Trail Mix (see page 264 for recipe)

1 glass of iced tea with lemon

1 med. orange

#### LUNCH:
Tempeh-Cucumber sandwich:
  2 slices whole-grain bread, toasted
  1/4 cup tempeh (packaged, cut into slices)
  4 to 6 slices of cucumber
  1 tbsp. reduced-fat Ranch dressing as spread
  sliced tomato and red onion

handful of baby carrots with 2 tbsp. humus dip

1 fresh peach

#### SNACK:
1 serving of Midnight Madness (see page 82 for recipe)

3 cups air-popped popcorn

#### DINNER:
1 cup marinara sauce made with fresh cut tomatoes served over

1 cup cooked pasta sprinkled with 1 ounce grated Parmesan cheese

1 cup steamed broccoli and pearl onions

1 whole-wheat sourdough bread dipped with 2 tsp. rosemary-flavored olive oil

1 serving Strawberry Cobbler (see page 262 for recipe)

**Nutritional Profile: Total Calories 2000 with 3 servings of soy**

Protein: 77 grams   Fat: 43 grams   Carbohydrate: 357 grams   Fiber: 44 grams

(or)

## Nutrition Facts

Serving Size 1 Day's menu

| Amount per Serving | |
|---|---|
| Calories 2000    387 Calories from fat | |
| | % Daily Value |
| Total Fat 43g | 66% |
| Saturated Fat 11g | 56% |
| Cholesterol 59mg | 20% |
| Sodium 2280mg | 95% |
| Total Carbohydrate 3575g | 119% |
| Dietary Fiber 44g | 177% |
| Protein 77g | |

Vitamin A 376%  •  Vitamin C 670%
Calcium 85%    •   Iron 135%
Folic Acid 110%  •  Vitamin E 230%

# *Eating Strategies That Fit Your Life*

Let's face it—knowing what to eat for a healthy heart is one thing, but doing it is another. We all face daily challenges that put us in a time crunch, and all too often, this puts good-for-you nutrition on the back burner. But following the Simple Six Eating Plan is truly *simple*. With the basics behind us, let's take a look at everyday situations. In this chapter, I show how to eat out—in restaurants and in fast-food outlets. And there's a simple guide to heart-healthy supermarket shopping to best stock your home with the easy-to-fix basics for the Simple Six.

## Eating on the Run—Using the Simple Six

### *Restaurant Dining*

If you find yourself eating food prepared outside your home about as often as you brush your teeth, join the millions of other American consumers who dine out. Some 30 years ago, the average consumer only spent 25 cents on every food dollar away from home. That was when eating out meant a special occasion. Today, according to food industry surveys, consumers spend about half of every food dollar on food prepared away from home.

The reason for this dining-out craze stems from lack of time. With couples, single parents, and working folks harried from the struggles of daily life, sitting down to a home cooked meal isn't happening as often as it used to. A food trends survey showed that 46 percent of the people eating out reported doing so because they had no time for cooking at home while only 5 percent reported dining out as a way to mark special occasions. Dining out has become a necessary survival technique.

But despite the "need" to dine at eating establishments, many people still view eating out as an opportunity to splurge. From larger portions, fatty sauces, and calorie-laden desserts, eating can easily take a toll on your heart health. Joan and Tom, a working couple with high-school-aged children, ate out at least two to three times per week out of necessity. I worked with them closely for a few weeks to scale down the amount of fat and calories in their diets. Both Joan and Tom commented they had no idea their dining-out routine (marked by large serving sizes, sauces with loads of hidden fat, and frequent desserts) was such a calorie and fat disaster.

Since eating away from home has become such an integral part of our daily lives, the food you select when dining out should help heal your heart and fit in the Simple Six Eating Plan. Use these basic dining-out tactics for heart-healthy eating in restaurants:

- *Before ordering, check the entire menu for healthful selections.* Many restaurants have sections on the menu that identify lower fat or heart-healthy entrées. Ask about daily specials that may also be prepared in ways that save on calories and fat.

- *Ask questions about how foods are prepared.* Many dining establishments will modify selections to your liking by cutting back on added oil and butter, or by grilling instead of frying.

- *Opt for sauces or dressing to be served on the side.* Often, most of the calories in a dish come from the rich sauce. Having it on the side lets you control the calories and fat.

- *Ask for substitutions or changes to your order.* Request that fresh fruit be substituted for hash browns with your morning eggs, or that fresh sliced tomatoes replace French fries with your lunch-time sandwich. These simple switches help boost your intake of vitamins, minerals, fiber, and phytochemicals that fight heart disease and high blood pressure while at the same time saving on calories and fat.

- *Ask for low-fat condiments for added flavor.* Many restaurants will happily provide upon request any number of condiments such as vinegar, specialty mustards, salsa, hot pepper sauce, or fresh ground pepper.

- *Control portion sizes.* If you know an eating establishment serves hefty portions, request a smaller one or plan on splitting your entrée with a friend. You can always take home leftovers that can be used as tomorrow's lunch.

### Fast Foods You Can Eat

"Fast foods you can eat" almost sounds like an oxymoron if you're concerned about heart health. Virtually every fast-food restaurant is noted for fatty and salty fare. From double-stacked burgers with special sauce to side salads smothered in creamy-rich dressings, escaping fat for your heart's health becomes a slippery challenge. And if you're watching sodium, you can easily exceed your daily allotment in one fast-food meal. But, eating with heart health in mind can be done. With some thought and a bit of preplanning, you can easily eat a meal at most fast-food eateries that fits into your Simple Six Eating Plan.

Let's start off with my Six Basic Rules of Fast-Food Restaurant Eating. Notice I call them "rules" rather than "tips." When it comes to fast-food outlets, if you enter those doors or drive up to that window armed with "rules," you are more apt to drive away with fast food that won't clog your arteries.

1. *Think control.* You are in charge of what you order. I say this because walking into a fast-food eatery and being overcome with the aroma of sizzling French fries weakens any soul with good intentions. So before you walk in, have a food-ordering plan. Waiting to see what "looks good" is a surefire way to end up with a fat disaster on your hands.

2. *Buy small.* With most chains now offering a "super deal" on "super sizing," it's hard to pass up that extra scoop of fries or larger burger. But usually the smallest item on the menu, the junior burger or plain taco for example, is the lowest in calories and fat.

3. *Pass on fried.* Frying foods such as potatoes (to make French fries), chicken, and fish add scads of unwanted fat calories. Opt for the grilled version where available. Request a baked potato (sans melted butter) instead of French fries. With the potato, you get a dose of heart-healthy fiber and vitamin C. Select a grilled chicken sandwich over fried chicken, either in pieces or in a sandwich.

4. *Skip the toppings.* A regular burger, side salad, and baked potato all start out relatively low in fat (or even fat-free, in the case of a salad or potato), but by the time spreads, dressing, and melted cheese and margarine make their way on top of these foods, you have a large dose of fat, typically artery-clogging saturated fat. Ask for toppings to be omitted or request them on the side so that you can apply a small amount for taste. Some eateries supply fat-free dressings if you request them.

5. *Go easy on drinks.* I am not referring here to alcoholic drinks but rather the sugared sodas and sweetened iced teas that add extra calories (albeit they are fat-free.) Watch serving sizes; some of the thirst-buster mega drinks pack over 500 calories (all from sugar.) Shakes are also a no-no unless you complement them with a low-fat item such as a side salad dressed with fat-free dressing. McDonald's milk shakes are under 30 percent fat calories, so on occasion they can make a great-tasting treat. Stick with water or diet sodas to quench your thirst, or opt for low-fat milk for extra nutrition at fast-food outlets.

6. *Ditch the desserts.* Fruit pies, sundaes, and the like are loaded with fat and not much of anything else. Your best bet is to bring along your own sweets such as fresh fruit or a fig cookie or two. Some fast-food outlets serve up frozen yogurt, which on occasion is okay, but ask yourself if you need the extra calories since most fast-food meals pack more than what you would have eaten at home.

## Supermarket Success: Simple Six Shopping Guide

We spend some $400 billion yearly in grocery stores. From fresh baked bread and rotisserie chicken to boxed cereals and canned chili, grocery stores average over 10,000 items. Additionally, in-store delis that now stock freshly prepared meals and side dishes for take-out have added a new dimension to grocery shopping. In fact, with their ready-to-eat offerings, supermarkets are cooking up some stiff competition for fast-food chains and local eateries who are after the same "on-the-go eater."

With so many products fighting for your attention, supermarket shopping has become an overwhelming task. But you can easily shop in this land of plenty with my Simple Six Shopping Guide.

### AISLE-BY-AISLE GUIDE

**Produce payoff:** Make your first stop in the store the produce section. Since you're eating at least eight servings of fruits and vegetables daily, park your cart here for fresh, heart-healing staples.

- *Look for color.* Buy an array of colorful fruits and vegetables—carrots, tomatoes, melons, berries, and more to get a variety of heart disease fighting phytochemicals.
- *Think packaged.* As a time saver, purchase packaged greens like spinach and collard greens (already cleaned). You will also find ready-cut veggies great for stir-fries or munching.
- *Go for variety.* Rather than sticking to the same vegetables and fruits, try new ones. Venture out and sample different types of mushrooms, for example, or hot peppers (if you like food spicy!).
- *Salads to go.* Ready-to-eat salads complete with fat-free or reduced-fat dressing in the bag are available in most grocery stores. You can also purchase shredded cabbage, great for coleslaw or stir-fries (see Cabbage in Part Two).
- *Find flavor in herbs.* Fresh herbs such as rosemary, basil, dill, and thyme, sold in bunches, are great for heart-healthy cooking (see Herbs in Part Two). They stay fresh in the fridge when stem ends are wrapped in a damp paper towel and kept in a plastic bag in the crisper drawer.

- *Buy bulk.* You can purchase dried fruits and nuts such as almonds and walnuts in bulk and use for trail mix and more (see Almonds and Walnuts in Part Two).

- *Look for ready-to-eat fruit.* If buying whole melons and other fruits seems like too much effort to prepare, you can purchase small containers of fresh fruit like melon and pineapple ready to eat.

- *Select soy.* Typically available in a refrigerated case located in the produce section is a wide array of tofu, baked tofu, tempeh and other soy foods including soy "hot dogs" and ground "meat" (textured soy protein). In time, you'll have your favorite brands of tasty soy foods.

**Meat and seafood market:**   Nothing like the meat counter of years ago, you'll find many time-saving and heart-healthy selections.

- *Fetch some fish.* Most supermarkets have a wide selection of fresh fish and other seafood packed with heart-healthy omega-3 fats (see Salmon and others in Part Two).

- *Look for precooked.* Sold in packages, precooked shrimp, chicken strips, and other meats are easy ingredients for a burrito, salad, or other dish.

- *Buy lean.* Look for *lean* cuts of beef (see Beef in Part Two), and other meats.

- *More ways to save time.* Purchase ready-to-cook filets of fish, chicken, or cuts of meat that have already been marinated. Broil in the oven or toss on the grill along with steamed vegetables; add fresh fruit and green salad to make a tasty meal.

**All that is canned, boxed, and bottled:**   Usually located in the center aisles of the supermarket is a dizzying array of kitchen staples from basic cans of beans and tomato sauce to packages of pasta salads and ready-to-munch snacks.

- *Get beaned.* Select at least three different types of canned beans, ready to use in soups, salads, and more (see Beans in Part Two). Choose from black beans, garbanzo, white beans, butter beans, and more; select low-sodium varieties if you are watching your sodium intake.

- *Buy meals in a can.* A great time saver (besides being heart-healthy) are the chili, soup, and bean dishes sold in a can. Vegetarian chili is my favorite and I always keep a selection of hearty soups that fix into a quick meal anytime. Be sure to pick up canned tuna, salmon, and clams for heart-healthy omega-3 fats.

- *Pick up staples.* Always keep your kitchen stocked with canned tomato products (sauce, chopped, seasoned), packaged pasta (look for whole grain), rice (brown is better—instant version saves time), bottles of olive and canola oil, vinegar, bottled salad dressings (reduced or fat-free), canned fruits packed in their own juice, and other staples such as whole oats and flour.

- *Read the box.* When selecting ready-to-eat cereals, look for those with plenty of fiber (see Breakfast Cereals in Part Two).

- *Second guess snack foods.* A savory selection of chips, crackers, and more await you, but before you buy, check the label for fat content (and sodium if you're on the lookout). There are many fat-free products that can fit in the Simple Six but man does not live by fat-free chip alone. (See Chips, Crackers, and other snack foods in Part Two.)

- *Think spicy.* Dried herbs and other seasonings are a must. Many new products such as herb blends take the guessing out of what flavorings go together.

**Dairy delights:** You'll notice there's more in the dairy case than milk these days.

- *Reach for nonfat.* Select fat-free milk (or 1%) and other dairy products. Stock up on plain and vanilla-flavored yogurt for eating and for use in recipes. Nonfat sour cream also makes a tasty garnish for burritos, chili, and curries.

- *Check out the cheeses.* Pick up Parmesan cheese for grating over pasta and steamed vegetables. Select reduced-fat cheeses for cooking and eating.

- *Don't go eggless.* Eggs fit into your diet, either whole eggs or egg substitutes, so be sure to keep some on hand. (See Eggs in Part Two.)

- *Find quick fixes.* Ready in minutes, packaged pasta dishes such as lobster ravioli or spinach tortellini, along with sauce, can be found in the dairy case. Before buying, check the label for unwanted fat.

**Bakery and deli:**   These supermarket sections are expanding daily with new offerings of freshly prepared foods designed to save you time. But look before eating; some come loaded with unwanted fat.

- *Reach for bread.* Most in-store bakeries bake bread daily. Basic sourdough bread, bagels, and the like are some of the tastiest low-fat foods (select whole grain when available).

- *Look out for muffins, cakes, and other treats.* Most of these goodies come with added fat, most often vegetable shortening with artery-clogging *trans* fats. Some bakeries may offer reduced-fat versions; ask questions about ingredients.

- *Sandwich sense.* Most deli sections sell packaged lunch fixings as well as custom-made sandwiches to go. Select fillings low in fat; many lunch meats such as Healthy Choice® come with under two grams of fat per 2-ounce serving.

- *Get to know sausages and other processed meats.* Before picking up a package of your favorite sausages or packaged whole ham, check out the label for fat, saturated fat, and sodium content. Most supermarkets offer a variety of tasty reduced-fat versions (reduced-sodium, too) of old-time favorites.

**Frozen wonderland:**   Last but not least the frozen food aisles are filled with take-home delights that quickly make up into heart-healthy meals and treats.

- *Think vegetables and fruits.* From spinach to soybeans, the frozen food aisle is awash with veggies to fill your Simple Six. Look for stir-fry ready vegetables (sometimes sold with a seasoning pack and noodles). You also find a selection of frozen berries, peaches, and other fruits that make great additions to smoothies and desserts.

- *Buy ready made.* Stock up on frozen dinners and entrées (see pages 146–147 for best picks), or look for family-sized vegetarian lasagna or other frozen meals that just take reheating before eating. Check the label for fat content.

- *Go fishing.* With the increase in demand, a large variety of ready-to-eat fish and seafood products are now available. Fish filets with no added fat and precooked shrimp, for example, can be ready in minutes.

- *Pause at pizza.* Frozen pizza can be a super pick or a disaster. Check the label for fat and saturated fat (see page 216 for a run-down).

- *Try ethnic.* Chinese stir-fries, Indian curries, and Thai spring rolls can be found in your frozen food case. Try out these and other ethnic entrées for variety.

- *Say soy.* Stock up on soy burgers, breakfast links, and other heart-healing soy foods from your freezer section. (See Soy in Part Two.)

### Dinner's Ready: In-Store Meals

Supermarkets across the U.S. have spent millions revamping their deli sections to include state-of-the-art cooking equipment, serving counters, soda dispensers, and even in-store seating for convenient dining. Some local markets cater more toward the gourmet dishes, serving specialty ethnic foods, fancy appetizers, and side dishes fit for entertaining. But most "supermarkets" are taking on a home-style restaurant look serving more traditional main meal offerings like meatloaf, chicken, and meatballs.

Here's a sampling of the meal menus from a variety of grocery stores along with the best picks and what's best left behind.

SALADS AND SIDE DISHES   You find the most variety in the salad and side dish section. For example, most Lucky Food Stores offer one to two dozen different cold salads from the basic potato salad to tri-colored pasta salad with fresh herbs and sundried tomatoes. Many supermarkets are now carrying at least one type of cold tofu salad that easily fits into your Simple Six Eating Plan. Ready-to-eat tofu salads are typically prepared with an ethnic flair such as Thai-spiced tofu with vegetables. Most salads are sold by the pound, but single-serve portions are available with dressing packed separately for freshness.

**Best picks:** Carrot salad (packed with heart-protecting carotenes), tomato (a source of another carotene called lycopene) and cucumber salad, three bean salad, and pasta salad with vegetables (broccoli, carrots, and red and green peppers) are good bets. Also include fruit salad made with melon, pineapple, berries, and grapes (loaded with potassium and vitamin C). Since recipes vary from store to store, ask about dressing ingredients and request that oily dressing be drained off or separated from your purchase. Good side dish choices include stuffed baked potatoes, roasted peppers filled with blended cooked veggies and bread crumbs, and vegetable quiche made without cream.

Some salads and side dishes come prepackaged. An array of packaged ethnic salads, for example, are available at many supermarkets. Some prepackaged salads also come with seasoned cubed tofu or tempeh. Try a Japanese salad made with soba noodles (made from wheat mugwort), shredded carrots, pea sprouts, nori, sesame seeds, and a tasty dressing. Each serving provides over 150 percent of the daily value for vitamin A, 40 percent for vitamin C, and 20 percent of iron needs. Or perhaps a Thai salad strikes your fancy, made from Napa cabbage, cappellini noodles, cilantro, and plenty of peppers giving each serving about 100 percent of the daily value for vitamins C and A.

**Worst picks:** Avoid salads drenched in mayonnaise like cole slaw, macaroni, potato, or seafood salads. As an alternative to your deli favorites, some stores now offer fat-free mayonnaise potato and macaroni salads. Pasta salads with added olives, meat cold cuts like salami or ham and glistening with oil can easily pack over 15 grams of fat (about 25 percent of the Daily Value). Keep away from meat wrapped olives, meat stuffed mushrooms, and flaky pastry triangles filled with cheese. If you like the looks of a salad or side dish but aren't sure about the ingredients—simply ask.

MAIN MEALS  Most major supermarket chains have their own in-house line of main entrées that easily fit into the Simple Six Eating Plan. Raley's Food Stores in California, for example, serve up main dishes called "Dinner Tonight."

**Best picks:** Rotisserie chicken, a staple at most supermarkets, eaten without the skin is relatively low in fat and makes for good leftovers easily used the next day for lunch or dinner. Hot pasta dishes served with vegetarian marinara sauce or a light meat sauce are other low-fat selections. Increasing in popularity at grocery stores is a selection of freshly made Chinese stir-fry dishes.

Stick with selections packed with vegetables, tofu, seafood, and lean meats that haven't been deep fried.

You can also select from a variety of other ethnic dishes such as enchiladas, tamales, vegetable frittata, yakatori chicken (spicy marinated chicken served on a stick), and Mediterranean wraps. Wraps, the latest ethnic food fad, consist of flat bread (similar to a thick tortilla) wrapped up with a mixture of beans, cooked grains, chopped vegetables, and spices. Fresh wraps taste great and pack a nutritional punch.

**Worst picks:** Unless the in-store chef assures you extra-lean cuts of meat are used, you're better off skipping the meat loaf, roasted pork tenderloin, and other traditionally fatty meats. Also, spicy chicken wings, fried chicken pieces, and heavy meatballs make for fat disasters. Check the warming pans for telltale signs of grease or fat drippings; this is a good sign you're better off leaving the food where it is.

# Abalone to Zucchini

*101 Miracle Foods
That Fit in the Simple Six*

Did you know that a cup of tea, a juicy orange, and a sinfully rich piece of chocolate all hold the key to a healthy heart? Many foods, even unsuspected foods such as beer and chocolate, may help you eat away the threat of heart disease and high blood pressure. Welcome to the world of Miracle Foods.

## A Guide to Miracle Foods

From Abalone to Zucchini, I compiled a list of powerful foods that eat away heart disease and high blood pressure. As you read, here's what to look for with each food.

### Simple Six Symbols

These symbols, the same ones used in Chapter Two, guide you in fitting each food into your eating plan.

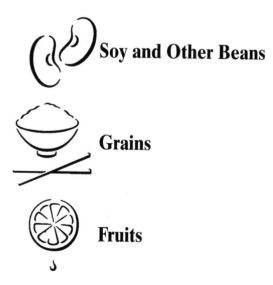

**Soy and Other Beans**

**Grains**

**Fruits**

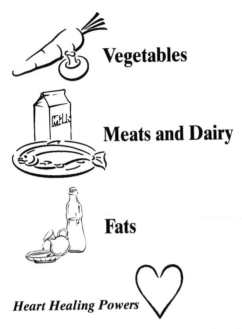

**Vegetables**

**Meats and Dairy**

**Fats**

*Heart Healing Powers*

Look for this icon on certain foods which indicates nutritional plusses, shown through scientific research, that help lower risk for heart disease, fight high blood pressure, lower blood cholesterol, or that offer some other heart-healing power. I also show you the research supporting and proving the power of each food.

*Food Profile*

For each food, I give you a rundown on its nutrition profile including calories per serving, fiber content, and key nutrients. Also, particular attention is paid to heart-disease fighting nutrients, phytochemicals, and more. I also include charts, graphs, and tables helpful for making comparisons with similar foods.

### *Food How-to's*

I provide you with selection, handling, and storing tips for each food, along with the best ways to prepare and serve it. I also pass along my favorite recipe and include the nutritional information using a food label for easy reading.

## Label Ease

Each recipe is followed by a partial food label. Here's a quick guide to make label reading easy.

|  | **Nutrition Facts** |
|---|---|
| **1.** | Orange 'n Bean Salad<br>Serving Size 1/6 recipe |
|  | Amount per Serving |
| **2.** | Calories 119    36 Calories from fat |
|  | % Daily Value* |
| **3.** | Total Fat 4g    6% |
| **4.** |   Saturated Fat <1g    2% |
| **5.** | Cholesterol 0mg    0% |
| **6.** | Sodium 301mg    13% |
| **7.** | Total Carbohydrate 20g    7%<br>  Dietary Fiber 4g    16% |
| **8.** | Protein 5g |
| **9.** | Vitamin A 1%  •  Vitamin C 48%<br>Calcium 4%  •  Iron 6% |

*Percent Daily Values are based on a 2000 calorie diet. Your daily values may be higher or lower depending on your calorie needs.

|  |  | Calories | 2000 | 2500 |
|---|---|---|---|---|
| **10.** | Total Fat | Less Than | 65g | 80g |
|  | Sat. Fat | Less Than | 20g | 25g |
|  | Cholesterol | Less Than | 300mg | 300mg |
|  | Sodium | Less Than | 2400mg | 2400mg |
|  | Total Carbohydrate | | 300g | 375g |
|  | Dietary Fiber | | 25g | 30g |

1. Use serving size guide in Chapter Two. All the nutrition information on the label is provided on a "per serving" basis and compared to a 2000 calorie diet (see bottom portion of label).

2. Compare with your calorie needs for the day.

3. Total fat per serving is measured in grams and is given a percentage comparison to the Daily Value, which is a daily fat "budget" of 65 grams.

4. Saturated fat is measured in grams, and compared by a percentage to the saturated fat Daily Value, which is 20 grams per day.

5. Cholesterol is measured in milligrams, and a percentage comparison is made to the daily allotment of 300 milligrams.

6. Sodium is measured in milligrams, and a percentage comparison is made to the daily limit of 2400 milligrams.

7. Dietary fiber is measured in grams, and a percentage comparison is made to the Daily Value of 25 grams.

8. Protein is also measured in grams. Your need varies from about 50 to about 80 grams, depending on body size. Using the Simple Six Eating Plan, you get about one-third of your protein from soy foods.

9. The percentage of your requirement is shown for key vitamins and minerals you are getting in this food.

10. I omit this standard portion of the label throughout the book since it merely lists general dietary standards for total fat, saturated fat, cholesterol, and others, and does not reflect nutritional information for the actual food or meal which is shown in the top portion of the label.

# Abalone

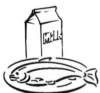

A delicacy dish at most seafood restaurants, this shellfish (when prepared heart-smart) makes a tasty addition to your Simple Six Plan. Technically a sea snail, abalone is both low in calories and low-fat: 85 calories per 3-ounce serving and less than a gram of fat, along with 15 grams of high-quality protein.

Many people stay away from abalone and other shellfish for fear of artery-clogging cholesterol. I have good news: Most of the 72 milligrams of "cholesterol" found in abalone is a look-alike substance called a *sterol* that can actually block cholesterol absorption in the digestive tract. So if you enjoy abalone, clams, and other shellfish, don't give the cholesterol another thought.

Abalone has even more to offer in the way of heart-healthy nutrition: a good dose of magnesium to help fight hypertension. Because of abalone's delicate texture and taste, there's no need for heavy cream sauces or deep-fat frying to doctor up the taste. Serve abalone cooked quickly in a nonstick skillet alongside fresh greens and a serving of wild-rice pilaf. (Go for the quick-cook grocery store version to save time.) At restaurants, ask that any accompanying sauce be put on lightly, or better, served on the side so you can control the amount. If you're lucky enough to have some fresh abalone at home, check out my recipe for Seafood Stew on page 119.

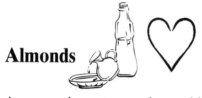

# Almonds

Are you going nuts over the nutritional advice on whether or not to eat nuts? I give you the bottom line: Most nuts, while packed with fat, have heart-healthy monounsaturated fat that won't put a glitch in your cholesterol reading. Almonds, in particular, are Mother Nature's heart-protecting nut. In every ounce, you get 10 percent of fiber and zinc needs, 25 percent of magnesium, and a good dose of vitamin E. Research shows that with the help of these nutrients, eating almonds as part of your daily fare can lower blood cholesterol levels.

In a recent study, researchers from Canada and the U.S. selected men and women with risky blood cholesterol levels as subjects for an almond eating study. For the first few weeks, the participants ate a heart-smart low-saturated fat, low-cholesterol, high-fiber diet that limited fatty meats, dairy products, and eggs.

For the next nine weeks all the participants ate 3 1/2 ounces of almonds daily and used only almond oil in cooking. This addition of almonds boosted the participants total intake of fat from 28 percent to a whopping 37 percent of total calories from fat, a level that's sure to send cholesterol levels skyrocketing. But most of the fat increase was from almonds' heart-healthy monounsaturated fats that have a quieting effect on blood fat levels.

Following the nine weeks of daily almond eating, researchers were pleased to discover that participants' average cholesterol levels dropped significantly, putting everyone's cholesterol levels out of the high-risk range. And more good news: LDL levels (that's the bad stuff), plummeted without a change in the cholesterol good guy, HDL. Researchers suspect that the positive effect of almonds may result from other key nutrients found in this heart-healthy snack, including vitamin E and fiber, in addition to the monounsaturated fats. Vitamin E, for example, helps protect LDLs from oxidizing, which stops these nasties from damaging artery walls.

Make almonds a regular part of your daily menu. Include a handful of almonds atop your morning whole-grain cereal or yogurt, or even blend them up in your favorite smoothie recipe. You can also use almonds to turn any ordinary green salad into a gourmet salad, or add to a fresh fruit medley for a refreshing crunchy flavor experience. My favorite is taking almonds with me anywhere as part of an energizing trail mix. This quick recipe can be easily doubled and stored in an airtight container in the fridge for a grab-anytime snack. When selecting almonds, buying bulk is less expensive (many supermarkets now sell almonds and other nuts in bulk) but make sure your food store has enough turnover to ensure that the nuts are fresh. Store almonds in the freezer or refrigerator; the cool temperatures keep the heart-healthy fats and vitamin E from breaking down.

### *Cran-Almond Trail Mix*

1 cup whole almonds
1 cup dried cranberries
1/2 cup raisins
1/4 cup dry-roasted pumpkin seeds

1/4 cup dried coconut (optional)

1/2 cup roasted soy nuts

Combine all ingredients and store in plastic container with a tightly-fitting lid. Trail mix keeps for six to eight weeks in the refrigerator. Makes about 10 one-third-cup servings.

| **Nutrition Facts** | |
|---|---|
| Cran-Almond Trail Mix | |
| Serving Size 1/3 cup | |
| Amount per Serving | |
| Calories 193 | 86 Calories from fat |
| | % Daily Value |
| Total Fat 10g | 15% |
|    Saturated Fat <1g | 4% |
| Cholesterol 0mg | 0% |
| Sodium 0mg | 0% |
| Total Carbohydrate 23g | 8% |
|    Dietary Fiber 3g | 13% |
| Protein 7g | |

| Vitamin A 0% | • Vitamin C <2% |
|---|---|
| Calcium 7% | • Iron 6% |
| | • Vitamin E 35% |

# Anchovy

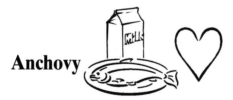

A favorite atop pizzas and in Caesar salads, anchovies come packed with heart-disease fighting goodies such as omega-3 fats, potassium, and calcium. A three-ounce serving of fresh anchovies has 110 calories and 4 grams of heart-healthy fat. And with each serving providing over 300 milligrams of potassium and 125 milligrams of calcium, two of the best high blood pressure fighting minerals, fresh anchovies are a stellar addition to your diet.

Know, though, that the canned variety, the type of anchovy you typically find on pizza and in salads, is packed in oil and comes crammed with over 700 milligrams of sodium in just five little anchovies—not good news if you're watching your sodium. If you're buying the canned variety for home use, make sure the anchovies are packed in fish oil (for extra omega-3) or olive oil, both good oils that don't push your blood cholesterol levels up. Canned anchovies also have a dose of calcium that does the heart good (as well as your bones).

Use canned anchovies as a garnish to homemade pizzas (topped with low-fat cheese) or add to your own version of Caesar salad using reduced-fat or nonfat dressing. Fresh anchovies can be used in soups, chowders, and stews. As with any fresh fish, store in the refrigerator for no more than two days or pop in the freezer wrapped tightly in freezer wrap for later use.

# Apples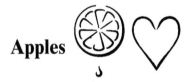

Eating an apple a day may very well keep heart disease away, according to several research studies. Modest by nutritional standards, apples supply little in the way of vitamins and only about five percent of potassium needs. But when it comes to fiber and phytochemicals, apples are outstanding. The fiber found in apples as well as other fruits, called *pectin,* has been shown to lower blood cholesterol. This same fiber is added to jellies, jams, and other foods as a thickening agent. In the intestines, pectin sweeps up and binds cholesterol keeping it from entering your system.

Researchers from Central Washington University put pectin to the test in people with mildly elevated blood cholesterol levels. For six weeks, a group of men drank apple juice supplemented with 10 grams of apple fiber while another group of men served as the control group and received an unsupplemented version of juice. At the end of six weeks, the apple fiber worked wonders.

Blood cholesterol levels fell an average of 10 percent in the group drinking the fiber-fortified juice. LDL levels fell a staggering 14 percent while HDL levels remained steady. These dramatic results from apple fiber are comparable to treatment with cholesterol-lowering drugs. That is solid evidence that apple fiber is a major player in the arsenal against heart disease.

There's more to the heart-healthy story for apples than fiber. While pectin found in apples effectively lowers blood cholesterol levels, other components of the apple may be just as beneficial. Research from the Netherlands found that elderly men who consumed a diet rich in the phytochemical group called *flavonoids,* specifically the type found in apples, had a lower risk of heart disease. In fact, those men who ate at least an apple a day cut their risk for dying of heart disease by 50 percent! These results certainly make a case for keeping a stockpile of apples on hand for munching.

Use apples as anytime snacks and heart-healthy desserts following lunch or dinner instead of fat-laced brownies or ice cream. You can also use apples in green salads for a crunchy sweet flavor, or try them in casseroles for a mildly sweet taste that complements your favorite recipe. Dried apples (make sure they come with the peel) can be eaten plain, added to trail mix, or cut into bite-sized pieces and used as a topper for your morning cereal or yogurt.

Applesauce still has the goodness of whole apples, especially when made with unpeeled apples. Check the label to see if peeled fruit was used. Even without the peel, apple pulp contains some pectin fiber. When selecting fresh apples, pick firm fruit without visible bruises or open marks. Apples stored in the fridge or a cold room can last up to a few weeks. Check out my recipe for Apple-Walnut Salad as a simple meal add-on that's great for your heart with the goodness of apples and walnuts (see Walnuts, on page 283).

### *Apple-Walnut Salad*

3 fresh apples (Red, Golden Delicious, or McIntosh work best)

1 carton nonfat vanilla yogurt

1/4 tsp. ground cinnamon

1/3 cup raisins

2 tsp. lemon juice

1/3 cup chopped walnuts

In a mixing bowl, stir together yogurt, cinnamon, raisins, lemon juice, and walnuts. Cut apples in quarters, and cut out core and seeds. Chop apple quarters into pieces about the size of small jelly beans. Stir apples into yogurt mixture. Chill briefly and serve garnished with mint leaves. Makes four servings.

| Nutrition Facts | |
| --- | --- |
| Apple-Walnut Salad | |
| Serving Size 1/4 recipe | |
| Amount per Serving | |
| Calories 230      60 Calories from fat | |
| | % Daily Value |
| Total Fat 6.5g | 10% |
| Saturated Fat <1g | 3% |
| Cholesterol 0mg | 0% |
| Sodium 45mg | 2% |
| Total Carbohydrate 41g | 14% |
| Dietary Fiber 5g | 20% |
| Protein 7g | |
| Vitamin A 1%   •   Vitamin C 19% | |
| Calcium 14%    •   Iron 6% | |

# Apticots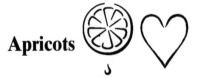

Whether you prefer fresh or dried apricots, you are sure to get a burst of beta carotene that, according to an array of research studies, protects your heart. Apricots also come with a good dose of potassium for fighting hypertension—over 300 milligrams, or 10 percent of your recommended daily intake in about three

## Carotene Count

Check out the carotene content of your favorite fruit.

| Fruit | Serving Size | Calories | Carotenes (milligrams) |
|---|---|---|---|
| Apricot, fresh | 3 whole | 54 | 1.3 |
| Apricot, dried | 10 halves | 83 | 6.0 |
| Cantaloupe | 1 cup pieces | 57 | 4.9 |
| Grapefruit | 1/2 medium | 37 | 1.6 |
| Guava | 1 medium | 45 | 0.7 |
| Mango | 1 medium | 135 | 2.6 |
| Papaya | 1 medium | 117 | 0.3 |
| Peaches, dried | 5 halves | 155 | 5.5 |
| Watermelon | 1 cup pieces | 50 | 6.9 |

*Source: Journal of the American Dietetic Association* 93: 284, 1993.

medium-sized fresh apricots. And at a mere 50 calories, a serving of this fresh fruit makes good heart sense. Dried apricots also pack a whopping 6 milligrams of beta carotene and 500 milligrams of potassium in 10 dried halves—all that with just 80 calories a serving.

Eating apricots and other fruits and vegetables rich in beta carotene may cut heart-disease risk, and the news is especially good for women. In an eight-year study involving over 87,000 women in the U.S., those women who regularly took in beta carotene rich foods had a 22 percent lower risk of heart disease than women who had a low intake. Other research studies that involve men also show this same heart-protecting effect of beta carotene. The bottom line for those on the heart watch: Keep apricots and other carotene-rich fruits and veggies a standard part of your daily eating routine. Check the "Carotene Count" chart for other great sources.

When buying fresh apricots, usually available during early summer, select firm fruit with a bright orange color (a little green is okay). Apricots ripen some in your kitchen fruit bowl, but re-frigerate soon so the fruit does not become overly ripe. Besides eating fresh, I like adding apricots to smoothies or chopping them into raisin-sized pieces to use as a topping for bagels or toast spread with light cream cheese. Dried apricots go anywhere: gym bag, worksite, or in your car for a super snack. And of course, you can always add chopped dried apricots to your favorite trail mix and use as a quick-energy and heart-smart snack.

## *Apricot-Cheese "Tartlets"*

10 fresh apricots

5 tbsp. part-skim ricotta cheese

1/2 cup brown sugar

1/2 cup almonds, chopped

Split each apricot (remove pit) and arrange halves in a glass baking dish. Fill each half with ricotta cheese and sprinkle about 1 tea-spoon of brown sugar on each half. Bake in a 375-degree oven for 20 minutes or until the brown sugar melts. Garnish with chopped almonds. Makes five servings. (I enjoy this topped with frozen, nonfat vanilla ice cream.)

## Nutrition Facts

Apricot-Cheese "Tartlets"

Serving Size 1 (2 whole apricots, filled)

| Amount per Serving | |
| --- | --- |
| Calories 214     74 Calories from fat | |
| | % Daily Value |
| Total Fat 8g | 13% |
| Saturated Fat 1g | 7% |
| Cholesterol 5mg | 2% |
| Sodium 28mg | 1% |
| Total Carbohydrate 33g | 11% |
| Dietary Fiber 3g | 12% |
| Protein 5g | |

| Vitamin A 23% | • | Vitamin C 12% |
| --- | --- | --- |
| Calcium 10% | • | Iron 9% |

# Artichoke

This vegetable is really a flower, and an immature one at that. An artichoke consists of leaf scales surrounding the edible "choke." On average, it takes 20 minutes to eat an artichoke, carefully scraping off the edible portion of the leaves. After all that work, your reward is a good dose of vitamin C, folate, and vitamin $B_6$ along with potassium. Both folate and vitamin $B_6$ help protect you from heart disease by clearing the blood factor, homocysteine, that can damage artery walls. The potassium works overtime in controlling high blood pressure.

Artichokes also contain a flavonoid called *silymarin.* This flavonoid, like those found in tea, onions, and other fruits and vegetables, acts as an antioxidant. This means silymarin protects against oxidative damage that can wreak havoc on LDLs, turning them into heart-disease time bombs.

Eating an artichoke is definitely worth the effort. Look for solid artichokes without scarred leaves. They keep a good seven to ten days in the refrigerator, sometimes more. Prepare artichokes by rinsing well in cold water. Then slice off tips of leaves and bottom stem if present. Put in a microwave-safe casserole dish with a lid, or in a covered pot on the stove. Microwave or steam until leaves pull out easily. Serve with a dip of freshly squeezed lemon juice mixed with fresh crushed garlic and a touch of heart-healthy olive oil. Or if you prefer a cream-type sauce, mix nonfat or reduced-fat mayonnaise with a spot of Worcestershire sauce and lemon.

What about those marinated artichoke hearts in a jar? Great on pizzas and in salads, but these are loaded with sodium and packaged in oil, so use them sparingly. Your heart will thank you for eating a freshly steamed artichoke.

# Asparagus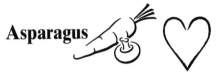

These mighty spears protect your heart with a natural source of the B-vitamin folate. Just a half-cup serving, about six spears cooked, contains 130 micrograms of folate—almost half the recommended daily intake, and over 140 milligrams of potassium, all for 22 calories. Quite a bargain considering folic acid helps protect your vessels from artery-damaging levels of the blood factor homocysteine.

As researchers unravel the mysteries of why heart disease develops in some individuals and not in others, homocysteine is turning out to be a major culprit in the process. Several studies suggest that high levels of homocysteine boost risk for heart disease and hypertension. Researchers theorize that as homocysteine levels climb, the blood vessels' elasticity, or stretchability, decreases—leading to scar tissue buildup simply from everyday blood movement.

So why is folate so important for nice stretchy blood vessels? This B vitamin is needed for normal metabolism as well as the clearance of homocysteine. A low intake of folate results in higher circulating levels of homocysteine, spelling trouble for blood vessels. Keep homocysteine levels in check by eating asparagus and other good sources of folate on a regular basis.

Asparagus, while best when in season during late winter and spring, can also be purchased frozen and is still a great source of folate. When selecting fresh asparagus, choose firm spears that don't appear shriveled at the end from dehydration. Since the tips are more tender, use in salads or lightly steamed as a side dish. The thicker, more pulpy stems can be cooked to a tender finish in soups or casseroles. Try my recipe for "Davis" California Rolls which pairs asparagus with ginger for a fresh flavor; see page 245.

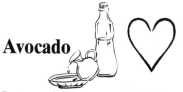

# Avocado

Let me change your mind about avocados. So often they top the lists of "bad" foods, but actually, avocados may even lower blood cholesterol. One medium Haas avocado (black bumpy type) has a whopping 340 calories, with over 70 percent coming from fat. But most of the fat is heart-smart monounsaturated. And according to a number of studies, an avocado-rich diet—about one to two a day—lowers artery-clogging LDL cholesterol. That is delicious news.

In one study, participants ate about one and a half avocados daily and their levels of LDL cholesterol dropped as much as when the subjects ate a low-fat, high carbohydrate diet designed by the American Heart Association to lower blood cholesterol. Other research showed that eating two avocados daily put fat intake at about half the total calories, yet significantly lowered total cholesterol, LDL, and blood fat levels. At the same time, levels of HDL, the "good" cholesterol, increased. This is good news considering the participants in this study had risky levels of cholesterol at the start.

Does this mean guacamole, an avocado lover's dream dip, should be a regular part of your diet? Certainly, enjoy it on occasion, but dieters beware. The extra calories from avocado should be balanced with a cut in fat elsewhere such as less salad dressing or oil used during cooking. Try my tried-and-true guacamole recipe dipped with fresh vegetables or fat-reduced chips. You can also use ripe avocados as a sandwich spread instead of mayonnaise or as a cream-cheese replacement on bagels.

### Guacamole with a Kick

2 ripe avocados (Haas)

1/2 cup nonfat sour cream

1/2 red onion, chopped

1 tomato, chopped

2 tbsp. cilantro, chopped

1/4 tsp. red pepper flakes

1 tsp. sesame oil

Mash avocados with a fork and blend in remaining ingredients. A food processor can be used if smoother consistency is desired. Refrigerate 30 minutes and serve with fresh vegetables or chips. Serves eight.

| **Nutrition Facts** | |
| :--- | ---: |
| Guacamole with a Kick | |
| Serving Size 1/8 recipe | |
| **Amount per Serving** | |
| Calories 122      63 Calories from fat | |
| | % Daily Value |
| Total Fat 7g | 11% |
| Saturated Fat 1g | 5% |
| Cholesterol 0mg | 0% |
| Sodium 40mg | 2% |
| Total Carbohydrate 13g | 4% |
| Dietary Fiber 4g | 16% |
| Protein 4g | |
| Vitamin A 8%   •   Vitamin C 19% | |
| Calcium 13%   •   Iron 4% | |

# Banana

Always a favorite, bananas seem to be a mainstay in fruit bowls in kitchens across the U.S. On average, we eat about 25 pounds of bananas per person every year. But what many of us don't realize is that this cool creamy tropical fruit helps protect the heart in two ways: First, the fiber found in banana pulp helps lower blood cholesterol and, secondly, the stockpile of potassium in a banana keeps blood pressure levels in check.

The type of fiber found in bananas is pectin—the same good stuff in apples and other fruit. In one study, researchers fed two groups of laboratory rats a diet loaded with fat and cholesterol that was sure to raise blood cholesterol levels. But one of the groups also ate banana pulp daily. Blood cholesterol levels fell in these rats despite the fact they were eating the equivalent of a burger-and-fries diet.

Fighting hypertension with a daily banana makes sense. One medium banana has about 450 milligrams of potassium, and in combination with the fiber, is an effective weapon against high blood pressure. Research shows that people who regularly eat fruit such as bananas take in more potassium and fiber and have a lower risk of hypertension. Bananas are also a good source of vitamin $B_6$ which plays a role in helping to break down damaging levels of the blood factor, homocysteine.

Good news for banana lovers: This fruit is available year round. Select green or slightly green bananas. They will ripen in a day or two at home. You can speed this up by putting bananas in a paper bag which traps the fruit-ripening gas called *ethylene*. Avoid putting bananas in the fridge as this turns their skin brown and stops the ripening process.

Snack on bananas anytime. There are only 110 calories in a medium banana. They work well in fresh fruit salad and the acid from other fruits such as oranges, strawberries, and melons helps keep banana slices from browning. Of course, my favorite way to eat a banana: Whip up one banana, two ice cubes, and a scoop of low-fat vanilla ice cream for a thick " 'naner" shake.

# Barley

Grain extraordinaire, barley can work wonders on your blood cholesterol levels. So far, researchers suspect that it's the fiber in barley in combination with small amounts of special fats found in the barley bran that help lower cholesterol levels. One cup of cooked pearled barley (outer tough layers removed) contains almost 10 grams of fiber. The fiber in barley is a mix of soluble fiber, known to lower blood cholesterol; and insoluble fiber, better known for keeping your intestines working regularly.

Researchers from Texas A&M University put barley bran and the oil from barley to the test in a group of men and women with high blood cholesterol levels. The study participants were put on a low-fat diet designed to help lower cholesterol levels. In addition, they were asked to add to their diets either barley bran flour or a few capsules of barley bran oil (extracted from barley bran) while a control group added a type of wheat fiber.

Following about a month of treatment, blood cholesterol levels dropped in those participants using barley bran flour or the barley oil. And more good news: Diastolic blood pressure also dropped significantly as a result of the diets. The researchers felt barley's cholesterol-busting action may have more to do with a special agent found in the barley bran oil than the actual fiber in the bran.

As for making barley a part of your regular menu, beer usually comes to mind, but this grain is actually very versatile. Hot cooked barley cereal topped with raisins makes a great warm start in the morning. For dinner, try mixing with onions and mushrooms for a pilaf-type side dish or use barley as a hearty addition to soups or stews for an evening meal.

Some supermarkets offer a quick-cook variety of barley that saves on the standard one-hour cooking time. I like using cooked barley in the same way as wheat bulgur. Next time you prepare barley, cook extra, refrigerate the leftovers, and try my Barley Salad recipe.

### Barley Salad

2 cups cooked barley, pearled

1 chopped tomato

1/2 med. cucumber, sliced then chopped

2 tbsp. chopped cilantro

1 tsp. chopped dill (use 1/4 tsp. dry dill if you don't have the fresh herb)

4 tbsp. olive oil/vinegar dressing (1:1 mix)

Mix all the ingredients together in a mixing bowl and serve. Use as a side dish for fish, grilled tofu, or sandwiches. Serves four.

## Nutrition Facts

Barley Salad

Serving Size 1/4 recipe

| Amount per Serving | |
|---|---|
| Calories 169     63 Calories from fat | |
| | % Daily Value |
| Total Fat 7g | 10% |
|    Saturated Fat 1g | 5% |
| Cholesterol 0mg | 0% |
| Sodium 6mg | 0% |
| Total Carbohydrate 25g | 8% |
|    Dietary Fiber 3g | 12% |
| Protein 2g | |

Vitamin A 3%   •   Vitamin C 13%
Calcium 2%   •   Iron 8%

# Beans—garbanzo, kidney, navy, white, and others

"Beans, beans, the magical fruit. The more you eat, the better it is for your heart." Perhaps a bit different from the rhyme you may remember, but more accurate. Beans are Mother Nature's wonder food when it comes to knocking down high blood cholesterol levels and protecting artery-clogging LDLs from damaging blood vessels. Countless research studies suggest that eating beans daily can have a "drug-like" effect on lowering blood cholesterol levels. And since beans, also called legumes, come in a wide variety and can be used in literally hundreds of different ways, you now have a great reason to make these power seeds part of your heart-smart Simple Six Eating Plan.

Beans' wonder ingredient is soluble fiber. Each half-cup cooked serving contains about one to three grams of soluble fiber, just shy of the soluble-fiber super food, oat bran. (See "The Magical Fruit Fiber Count" chart.) Famed fiber researcher James

## The Magical Fruit Fiber Count

| Bean (1/2 cup serving) | Calories | Total Fiber (grams) |
| --- | --- | --- |
| Black | 113 | 7.5 |
| Chickpeas | 134 | 6.2 |
| Kidney | 113 | 6.5 |
| Lentils | 115 | 7.8 |
| Lima | 96 | 6.8 |
| Navy | 129 | 5.8 |
| Peas, split | 115 | 8.1 |
| Pinto | 117 | 7.3 |
| White | 124 | 5.6 |

*Source:* Manufacturers' Food Labels and Bowes & Church's *Food Values of Portions Commonly Used*, 17th ed., Lippincott, 1998.

Anderson, M.D., has conducted several studies touting beans' benefits. In fact, studies show cholesterol levels are lowered over 20 percent following a daily dose of 1 1/2 cups of beans. Other studies show that beans push down LDL levels while helping boost levels of the cholesterol good guys, HDLs.

In addition to the fiber, beans also provide a hefty dose of heart-disease fighting folic acid and potassium, and each serving has about the same amount of protein as a glass of milk. Beans are also a great calorie bargain considering a serving contains a little over 100 calories and has only a speck of fat. Soybeans and peanuts, on the other hand, which are both technically beans or legumes, contain more fat. As you know from the Simple Six Eating Plan, soybeans have special heart-protecting powers. You can check out more on soybeans by turning to page 249, and for peanuts' benefits, see page 211.

And there's even more. Beans have special substances called *flavonoids* to help protect the heart in a powerful way. Flavonoids keep the LDLs, carriers of cholesterol, from becoming ornery and damaging artery walls. This type of protection is crucial to all of us looking to prevent heart disease or the development of new lesions in our blood vessels.

For most people, the thought of eating beans on a regular basis brings to mind two things: Time needed to soak and cook the beans, and well, gas. Good news: There is a way around both of these problems. Reach for the canned beans which are virtually identical in soluble fiber content to beans cooked the old-fashioned way. And trust me, the old-fashioned way takes time you may not have: Dry beans must be soaked overnight to soften, and then boiled for one to two hours. I prefer the 15-second version of opening a can of precooked beans. Canned beans come in many varieties that can be combined in bean dishes like chili and soup, so you're not limited by the convenience of a can. In the "Hill of Beans" chart, I list a variety of ready-made bean dishes that come in a can.

As for the gas, beans contain some indigestible carbohydrate that your large intestine bacteria munch on and make whoopee, and in doing so, form gas. As you eat beans more regularly, the gas problem subsides a bit. If you shy away from beans because of the gas problem, there is a solution—Beano®. Put a few drops of this tasteless "gas treatment" on your beans and a special enzyme in Beano® goes to work breaking down the indigestible carbohydrates that would have fed the gas-producing bacteria in your intestines. Hence, no more gas production.

### Bean Cuisine

I've never met a bean I didn't like. They can be used in so many ways, and beans are simple to store without the risk of going bad. Dry beans stored in airtight containers can last a year or so and canned beans (as long as you have the space) last a good couple of years in the pantry. Prepare dry beans by soaking in water overnight, drain the water, and then cook until tender in just enough water to cover them (this limited process helps reduce the level of the gas-forming carbohydrates). Or, you can use a short-cut method to soaking: Bring dry beans to a boil and then let them stand for an hour or two to soften before cooking.

Try cooked beans in cold salads as a topping, or make a bean salad by combining a few varieties, tossing with chopped tomatoes and scallions, and topping with bottled fat-free Italian dressing.

## Hill of Beans

Try out these high-fiber, low-fat, beans-in-a-can meals.

| | Serving Size | Calories | Fat (gm) | Protein (gm) | Fiber (gm) |
|---|---|---|---|---|---|
| *Soups* | | | | | |
| Campbell's Split Pea 'n Ham | 1 cup | 190 | 3 | 14 | 3 |
| Progresso Hearty Black Bean | 1 cup | 170 | 3 | 10 | 5 |
| Progresso Lentil | 1 cup | 140 | 1.5 | 10 | 8 |
| *Chiles* | | | | | |
| Dennison's 99% fat-free with beef | 1 cup | 220 | 2 | 22 | 6 |
| Nally with beef | 1 cup | 260 | 7 | 19 | 10 |
| Stagg with beef | 1 cup | 330 | 15 | 18 | 14 |
| Hormel 99% fat-free vegetarian | 1 cup | 200 | 1 | 12 | 7 |
| *Side Dishes* | | | | | |
| Campbell's Pork and Beans | 1/2 cup | 130 | 2 | 5 | 6 |
| Bush Baked Beans | 1/2 cup | 150 | 1 | 7 | 7 |
| Rosarita Refried Beans | 1/2 cup | 100 | 2 | 6 | 6 |
| Rosarita Vegetarian Refried Beans | 1/2 cup | 100 | 2 | 6 | 6 |
| Rosarita Nonfat Refried Beans | 1/2 cup | 90 | 0 | 6 | 2 |
| Green Giant Three-Bean Salad | 1/2 cup | 70 | 0 | 2 | 3 |
| Hummus (ground chickpeas) | 2 tbsp. | 60 | 3.5 | 2 | 1 |

*Source:* Manufacturers' Food Labels

Add beans to pasta or combine with cooked rice or other grain for a cholesterol-busting meal. Beans also make a hearty addition to casseroles, soups, and stews, and as fillings for burritos and wraps. They also stand alone as an excellent side dish with grilled fish or tofu.

### Black Bean Salad

1 can black beans, drained
1 can small red beans (kidney beans will do), drained
1 cup frozen or canned corn, drained
1/2 cup red onion, chopped
1/2 cup chopped fresh coriander
2 large tomatoes, chopped
ground pepper to taste

Mix all ingredients in a bowl. Optional: Add dried chili flakes to taste. Refrigerate one hour and serve as side dish or as an appetizer with fresh vegetables or reduced-fat corn or tortilla chips for dipping. Makes eight servings.

| **Nutrition Facts** |  |
| --- | --- |
| Black Bean Salad |  |
| Serving Size 1/8 recipe |  |
| **Amount per Serving** |  |
| Calories 83 | 5 Calories from fat |
| | % Daily Value |
| Total Fat <1g | 1% |
| Saturated Fat 0g | 0% |
| Cholesterol 0mg | 0% |
| Sodium 70mg | 3% |
| Total Carbohydrate 16g | 5% |
| Dietary Fiber 5g | 20% |
| Protein 5g | |
| Vitamin A 3% • Vitamin C 14% | |
| Calcium 2% • Iron 8% | |
| • Folate 20% | |

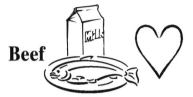

# Beef

Where's the beef? Anyone making a whole-hearted effort to keep their arteries unclogged may swear off eating beef altogether, or keep those juicy indulgences to "rare" occasions. But going beef-less is not a necessary step to stave off heart disease. In fact, studies show that beef, lean beef that is, does not cause heart disease. But there's a catch to this statement. Choose the right beef cuts, control the amount of beef, and prepare beef in a heart-smart way, and you can easily make lean beef a part of your Simple Six Eating Plan.

### *What's the Beef About Beef?*

Beef's bad rap primarily has to do with its high fat content. More importantly, a fair chunk of beef's fat is artery-clogging saturated fat. As a result, many heart-conscious people moved over to chicken as a lower-fat meat option. That move may have been based more on feeling than fact since several cuts of beef actually have less fat and less saturated fat than a skinless chicken thigh. As you can see from the "Beef Up" chart, top round, round tip, and top sirloin each have about a third less total fat than a chicken thigh (without the skin) as well as less saturated fat. Not all cuts of beef are this low in fat; compare the fat content of ribs and regular ground beef.

Studies show that beef itself, that is, minus the beef fat, is not damaging to the heart. In one study, a group of five men and five women ate 17 ounces of very lean beef (a lean cut such as top sir-loin with the visible fat trimmed away) every day for five weeks. Despite this beef fest, blood cholesterol levels dropped by nine percent compared to initial levels. When the researchers added back beef fat (as drippings) to the diet, blood cholesterol level rose dramatically. This suggests that beef (sans fat) is not the culprit but instead it's the fat on beef that poses a risk to your heart.

### *Beef or Chicken?*

So what will it be, beef or chicken? As part of a low-fat diet, lean beef appears to be as effective as chicken in lowering blood

## Beef Up

How chicken and beef compared on total fat and saturated fat in a 3-ounce serving (information listed in grams)

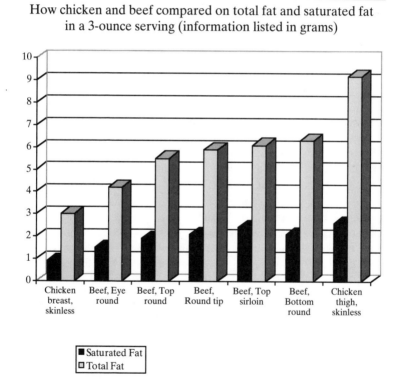

cholesterol levels. Researchers from the Baylor College of Medicine put subjects on one of two diets that were both low in fat, with either three ounces of cooked chicken or three ounces of cooked lean beef daily. Following five weeks, blood cholesterol levels dropped in both groups, and by the same amount, compared to prediet levels.

The beef versus chicken story goes beyond fat content. Some people who opt for chicken over beef feel they are dodging the cholesterol in red meat. But ounce for ounce, chicken and beef have the same amount of cholesterol—about 70 milligrams per three-ounce serving, cooked. If you've been advised by a physician to cut back on cholesterol, know that a serving of beef, chicken, or fish for that matter supplies a little less than 25 percent of your daily 300 milligram allotment.

### How Much Beef Is Okay?

Before I give you the bottom line on how much beef fits into your Simple Six Eating Plan, it's good to have some background on meat guidelines. Recommendations from the experts vary as to how much lean beef fits in a heart-healthy diet. Some proponents of a very low-fat diet designed to halt and even reverse heart disease, Dr. Dean Ornish, for example, advise a vegetarian or meatless cuisine. The American Heart Association recommends eating a diet low in fat, saturated fat, and cholesterol, but does not specifically advise on the red meat issue. The Food Guide Pyramid (that triangle-shaped food guide you see on a box of cereal and elsewhere) allows about five to seven ounces of meat daily.

Your choice to include beef in your diet should be based on other aspects of your daily food plan. Lean beef is a stellar source of other key nutrients that at times people may be lacking in their diets. For example, beef is a great source of the minerals zinc, crucial for a strong immune system, and iron, necessary for healthy circulation. Studies show that some people who avoid meat typically have poor intake of these minerals. That's not to say that you couldn't get these minerals from other food sources, it just so happens that many people fall short because they fail to make up the difference with other food.

A team of researchers heading the Bogalusa Heart Study from Tulane School of Public Health in New Orleans collected diet information from over 500 young adults. Those individuals eating six to seven ounces of meat daily had a better intake of zinc and other nutrients compared to those who had little meat in their diet. Also, the researchers noted no difference in heart-disease risk profile in the meat-lovers compared to those who ate very little.

Now for the bottom line on how much beef is okay. As you put together your Simple Six Eating Plan to fit your needs, keep in mind you are aiming for about two servings of soy products a day. Since soy, like beef, is a great source of protein, you needn't overemphasize beef as a means to meet your protein needs. Use two to four, three-ounce servings of beef per week as your guide. At this level, you have room for soy products, beans, fish, yogurt, cheese and other great sources of protein with heart-disease fighting powers.

### Beef Fixins'

Properly preparing beef is important not only for heart-healthy eating but for food safety reasons as well. Like all raw meats, handling and cooking beef properly can assist in averting food poisoning risk. When selecting beef, make sure to choose leaner cuts (see chart). At the meat counter you can ask for (or it should be on display) nutrition information on various cuts of beef and other meats. Store meat in the refrigerator if you will be using it within a day or two, or to keep longer, freeze beef in proper wrapping such as a freezer bag (it keeps for about 4 months).

Before cooking beef, trim all visible fat. The best cooking method for beef depends on the cut. For more tender cuts such as top sirloin, use grilling, roasting in the oven, or pan broiling (in a nonstick skillet) as cooking methods. Tougher cuts including top round require slower methods that use moisture or water such as stewing or adding to soups. Also, soaking in a marinade helps tenderize the meat.

Beef's versatility makes it a great addition to all types of dishes. Due to its flavor, especially if marinated beforehand, a small amount goes a long way. Remember that a three-ounce serving is the size of a deck of cards. Quick-cook thin strips of beef and add to a stir-fry of vegetables. Add small chunks of braised top round to a hearty carrot and potato stew. Stir in marinated beef strips into cooked black beans and use as a burrito filling (salsa is a must). Grill vegetables such as squash, tomatoes, and onions on a skewer with small pieces of top sirloin. Serve chilled bits of grilled top sirloin in pasta or green salad. Or simply grill a small sirloin steak and serve with brown rice pilaf, steamed vegetables, and herbs along with a hunk of whole-grain sourdough bread for a tasty and heart-healthy meal. Since I enjoy grilling when the weather permits, veggie-beef kabobs are one of my summertime favorites. The peppers in this recipe pack heart-disease fighting phytochemicals.

### Red-Yellow-Green Beef Kebobs

1 pound of beef sirloin steak (no bone), cut into 1 1/2-inch cubes

1 tbsp. olive oil

1 tsp. sesame oil

1 tbsp. lime juice

1 tbsp. balsamic vinegar

1 tsp. crushed garlic

1/4 tsp. ground pepper

1 each: red, yellow, and green bell pepper, seeded and cut into inch wide strips, then cut into squares

Combine oils, lime juice, vinegar, garlic, and pepper into a bowl. Add beef, stir to coat and let sit at least 30 minutes. Thread beef cubes and peppers onto four skewers. Start with peppers, using one of each color and alternate with beef. Place filled skewers on hot grill and cook about 12 minutes, turning until meat is done. Makes four servings.

## Nutrition Facts

Red-Yellow-Green Beef Kebobs
Serving Size 1 skewer

| Amount per Serving | |
|---|---|
| Calories 291     123 Calories from fat | |
| | % Daily Value |
| Total Fat 14g | 21% |
| Saturated Fat 4g | 21% |
| Cholesterol 101mg | 34% |
| Sodium 77mg | 3% |
| Total Carbohydrate 6g | 2% |
| Dietary Fiber 1g | 5% |
| Protein 35g | |

| | | |
|---|---|---|
| Vitamin A 5% | • | Vitamin C 114% |
| Calcium 2% | • | Iron 23% |
| Zinc 50% | • | Vitamin B$_{12}$ 54% |

## Play It Safe

Here are a few tips on handling and cooking beef to avert any run-ins with potentially harmful food bugs.

- *Thaw frozen beef in the refrigerator.* Bacteria can get hold of food when thawed at room temperature so that when you improperly handle the meat later, the risk of food poisoning is there.

- *Clean your cutting board well after handling raw meat.* It's a toss up whether wood or plastic is best—both can harbor bacteria. Use soap and warm water for cleaning. Better yet, keep one board for produce and another for meats (still clean after every use).

- *Wash your hands before and after handling raw meats.* Use soapy water and rinse well. Touching raw meat and then handling produce without washing is a kitchen taboo.

- *Cook beef to an internal temperature of 160 to 165 degrees.* This ensures that contaminating bacteria such as *E. Coli* gets zapped. This becomes particularly important when cooking ground beef. (Make sure it is super lean, typically made from ground top sirloin.) Cooking ground beef properly means that no pink color remains in the middle and that juices run clear rather than pink.

# Beer ♡

Ancient civilizations way back in about 5000 B.C. stumbled onto something: fermented wheat and barley. Realizing that this was something good, people recorded it; the world's oldest known recipe, scribbled on a 4000-year-old Sumerian tablet, is for beer. As part of our heritage, beer is in a sense a dietary staple. But when it comes to heart health, beer should be viewed as a "good-news-bad-news" food.

First, the good news: If drinking is kept "light" or moderate, the equivalent of one to two beers a day, studies show that alcohol has a protective effect against heart disease. Alcohol's benefit seems to be in raising the cholesterol good-guy HDLs which help scavenge and eventually remove cholesterol from the body. But since women already have higher HDL levels than men, the protective action of alcohol seems to be more beneficial for men.

The news for beer gets even better. Because beer is made from fermented grains, some phytochemicals called *flavonoids* end up in a bottle of beer. These flavonoids are similar to the heart-healthy phytochemicals found in red wine. According to heart researchers, flavonoids keep blood cells called *platelets* from becoming sticky and clumping together to form a clot, risking heart attack or stroke. Flavonoids found in beer also help protect artery-clogging LDLs from damaging blood vessel walls. Flavonoid content of beers varies. Dark beers have more pigment, owing to a higher flavonoid content. Lagers or lighter beers contain less.

Now for the bad news: Beer contains alcohol—about half an ounce in a 12-ounce, 150-calorie serving. Alcohol spells trouble for those concerned about hypertension. Research studies clearly show that alcohol intake is directly associated with high blood pressure. People who consistently drink six or more drinks daily have a greatly increased risk of suffering from hypertension. Heavy drinking also aggravates blood pressure in people who already have hypertension.

So is beer a heart-healthy drink? If you keep beer drinking in moderation (one to two drinks a day) and don't already have hypertension, go for it. But keep in mind that drinking any alcoholic beverage to excess has its risks, such as driving under the influence and operating machinery while intoxicated. Additionally, excessive alcohol can also increase risks for certain cancers, especially in women who also don't seem to gain much heart-health benefit from alcohol in the first place.

# Bell Peppers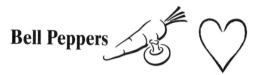

For starters, bell peppers come in an array of colors that are sure to liven up any plate. And it's their color—yellow, orange, red, green, and even purple—that determines the extent of their heart-protecting powers. Bell peppers pack a good dose of the antioxidants vitamin C and carotenes, and research shows these antioxidants work together in protecting the heart. Specifically, vitamin C and the carotenes found in bell peppers, lutein and zeaxanthin, help to keep LDLs from becoming a menace to blood vessels.

Depending on a pepper's color, the content of this antioxidant team varies. As a pepper ripens, it may change from green to red for example, and the vitamin C content increases along with the carotene levels. One green bell pepper contains about 140 percent of the Daily Value for vitamin C, but a red pepper has a whopping 280 percent. That's not bad for only 30 calories per serving. The content of the carotenes, lutein and zeaxanthin, goes up nine times as the pepper changes color. Yellow and orange peppers, along with purple, also have carotenes that protect the heart. In general, the more intense and brilliant the color, the better.

Bell peppers are best eaten raw for maximum vitamin C and carotene content. But since they're so rich in these nutrients, cooking peppers, such as baking or microwaving, still leaves behind plenty of heart-healthy goodness. Use a mix of freshly sliced peppers as a dipper for your favorite low-fat dip or in salsa. Grilled peppers make a great addition to fish, chicken, lean beef, or grilled tofu. Or try my All Red Salad as a refreshing side dish that is exploding with heart-healthy carotenes.

## All Red Salad

1 red pepper

1/4 head of red cabbage

1/2 sweet red onion

1 red apple

2 tbsp. balsamic vinegar

1 tbsp. olive oil

fresh ground pepper to taste

Cut pepper in half, clean out seeds, and slice into thin strips (width wise). Slice the cabbage and red onion into similar size slices. In a bowl, whisk oil and vinegar together. Toss in peppers, cabbage, and onion slices. Chill one hour. Before serving, slice apple into thin strips, toss lightly into the salad, and top with fresh ground pepper. Makes four servings.

| **Nutrition Facts** | |
| :--- | ---: |
| All Red Salad | |
| Serving Size 1/4 recipe | |
| **Amount per Serving** | |
| Calories 80    33 Calories from fat | |
| | % Daily Value |
| Total Fat 4g | 9% |
|    Saturated Fat <1g | 6% |
| Cholesterol 0mg | 0% |
| Sodium 5mg | 0% |
| Total Carbohydrate 13g | 4% |
|    Dietary Fiber 2g | 10% |
| Protein 1g | |
| Vitamin A 13%  •  Vitamin C 100% | |
| Calcium 3%  •  Iron 2% | |

# Berries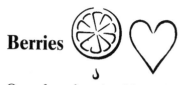

One of my favorite things about late spring and early summer is fresh berries topped lightly with whipped cream. While the cream might not be the greatest for heart health (I indulge every so often), the berries make up for it. Raspberries, blackberries, and marionberries, from the caneberry family, are loaded with vitamin C, cholesterol-lowering fiber, and an array of phytochemicals that help protect the heart.

One cup of fresh berries (actually two servings, because who can eat just half a cup?) packs over six grams of fiber. The type of fiber in berries is the water-soluble kind called *pectin.* Studies show that pectin helps lower blood cholesterol levels by soaking up cholesterol by-products in the intestinal tract and carrying them out of the body. This powerful pectin action effectively puts a damper on circulating cholesterol levels without actually getting *inside* the body. (I consider anything in your intestinal tract, start to finish, outside your body.)

In addition to fiber, berries supply vitamin C which helps protect blood vessels from the damaging LDLs. A one-cup serving has about 50 percent of the Daily Value for vitamin C. Also helping to protect your heart are a variety of phytochemicals in berries that have been shown to inhibit cholesterol production and in turn, lower blood cholesterol levels. One particular phytochemical group found in berries, called *catechins,* is also found in green tea and is responsible for the health benefits associated with this beverage.

Thanks to hot-house farming and imported produce, you can get berries year round, though sometimes pricey. And since berries only last a few days in the refrigerator, think frozen. You can get the same health benefits of fresh berries in the frozen version. This way, you can keep berries on hand for use in cobblers, topping for nonfat frozen yogurt, and your morning cereal. My standard routine is to always keep a bag of frozen raspberries and blackberries on hand to make up a fruit shake anytime. My Midnight Madness smoothie packs berry goodness along with the powers of soy protein.

### Midnight Madness

2 cups fresh or frozen blackberries (1/2 blueberries okay)

1 scoop (1/2 cup) frozen, nonfat vanilla ice cream or frozen yogurt

5 ice cubes

1 oz. (1 scoop) Health Source® soy protein powder, nonflavored

2 tsp. honey

3/4 cup skim milk

In a blender, combine all the ingredients, put the lid on, and blend on high until smooth. Makes two servings (one serving equals one soy serving).

| Nutrition Facts | |
|---|---|
| Midnight Madness | |
| Serving Size 1/2 recipe | |
| **Amount per Serving** | |
| Calories 222 | 9 Calories from fat |
| | % Daily Value |
| Total Fat 1g | 2% |
| Saturated Fat 0g | 0% |
| Cholesterol 5mg | 2% |
| Sodium 212mg | 9% |
| Total Carbohydrate 37g | 12% |
| Dietary Fiber 10g | 39% |
| Protein 18g | |
| Vitamin A 22% • Vitamin C 65% | |
| Calcium 34% • Iron 17% | |
| Vitamin $B_6$ 19% • Folate 27% | |

# Brazil Nuts

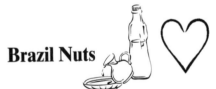

At first glance, these nuts hardly look like a heart-smart food. You know the ones I'm talking about—those few, big nuts in the mixed-nut bowl. One ounce, about eight medium brazil nuts, has 186 calories with a staggering 90 percent from fat! But look a little deeper into that fatty nut meat and you find a very special mineral called *selenium*. Brazil nuts happen to be the best source around of this special nutrient, containing over 25 percent of the requirement per serving. Research shows selenium may protect blood vessels from damaging cholesterol and reduce risk of heart disease.

Selenium's role as a heart protector comes from its work as an activator of a special enzyme called *glutathione peroxidase.* This enzyme puts a halt to any oxidative damage that makes the LDLs the "bad" cholesterol carriers in the circulation. If LDLs become oxidized, they eventually damage artery walls leading to fatty buildup and messy blockage. Skimping on selenium intake, found in meats and seafood as well as Brazil nuts and even drinking water, can put you at risk for heart disease.

In fact, in a small town in Northern Italy, scientists tracked the number of deaths from heart disease and found a direct correlation to the level of selenium in the town's drinking water. Selenium levels in all drinking water naturally fluctuate depending on rainfall and the selenium content of the surrounding soil. In the study, when selenium levels in the water supply fell over a several year period, the town's people took in less of this mineral, and the number of fatal heart attacks rose compared to other time periods when water selenium levels were greater. Plenty of other research shows that low circulating levels of selenium in our bodies is associated with greater risk of heart disease. You get the picture: Selenium is important for a healthy heart.

You can easily fit Brazil nuts in as part of your Simple Six Eating Plan. But dieter beware: Brazil nuts are high in calorie and fat content, so eating more than a handful or two may be more calories than you bargained for. Bottom line: Eat Brazil nuts in moderation, and your heart will thank you for it.

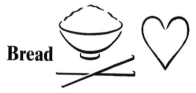

# Bread

No matter how you slice it, bread is good food. And it's good for your heart, too. Since Biblical times, bread has been synonymous with nourishment. Virtually all cultures around the world have some form of bread as a dietary staple. Bread made from grains such as wheat, rye, barley and oats supplies an array of nutrients that warm your heart with good health.

A slice of bread averages about 70 calories and packs a good dose of carbohydrates, iron, and B vitamins including folate, all with very little fat. The Food and Drug Administration's 1998 ruling that all processed grains must be fortified with folate helps ensure that more Americans get the heart protection this B vitamin provides. The added advantage of whole-grain breads such as 100 percent whole-wheat or whole-oat bread is their supply of vitamin E, other minerals including zinc, and even disease-fighting phytochemicals. (Check out the "By the Slice" chart for more nutrition info on breads.)

Bread's nutritional goodness may help explain why countries, including Italy and France, that fill their plates with bread and other grains have a lower risk for heart disease compared to the U.S. In Europe, people eat more carbohydrates, including bread, than people do in the U.S.: 55 percent of Europeans' total daily calories come from carbohydrates versus 45 percent in the U.S. And it's those high-carbohydrate diets that focus on whole grains, vegetables, and fruits, rather than fat, that have been shown to lower heart-disease risk.

Bread in particular may have heart-protecting powers. A study that included over 31,000 participants found that those regularly eating whole-wheat bread had about half the risk of a heart attack compared to those who ate very little. The protective ingredient in whole-wheat bread may be the fiber. Grains such as oats and barley have water-soluble fiber which is known to help lower blood cholesterol. Wheat fiber, while better at keeping your digestive system moving, may also have cholesterol lowering benefits.

Phytochemicals, special substances in grains, fruits, and vegetables that help fight disease, may also help protect your heart. Grains contain phenolic compounds, similar to the heart-healthy phytochemicals found in grape skins and red wine, which may help ward off heart disease. When whole grains are processed to make white flour, the outer hull of the wheat or grain kernel is removed. This process also strips the grain of these precious phytochemicals. Make an effort to select whole-grain breads and other grain products for heart health.

### Breaking Bread

From a basic loaf to a sophisticated English muffin, many bread "opportunities" await you. Following the Simple Six Eating Plan, your goal is approximately seven to eight servings of grain

## By the Slice

Here's how breads, bagels, muffins, and biscuits compare.
Note that serving sizes vary.

| Breads | Serving Size | Calories | Fiber (gm) | Carbo-hydrates (gm) | Fat (gm) |
|---|---|---|---|---|---|
| White, sourdough | 1 slice (1 oz) | 70 | 1 | 12 | 1 |
| Whole wheat | 1 slice (1 oz) | 61 | 1.6 | 12 | 1 |
| Rye | 1 slice (1 oz) | 80 | 2 | 15 | 1 |
| Multi-grain | 1 slice (1 oz) | 65 | 1.8 | 12 | 1 |
| Bagel | 2 oz | 150 | 1 | 30 | 1 |
| English muffin | 2 oz | 130 | 1 | 25 | 1 |
| Pita | 2 oz | 160 | 1 | 32 | 2 |
| Tortilla, flour | 2 oz | 160 | 1 | 25 | 4 |
| Biscuit | 1 oz | 93 | 0 | 13.6 | 3.3 |
| Muffin, blueberry | 1.5 oz | 126 | 1 | 19.5 | 4.3 |
| Muffin, bran | 2 oz | 183 | 3.9 | 31 | 5 |
| Scone, raisin | 1.5 oz | 229 | 1 | 30 | 10 |
| Croissant | 1 oz | 117 | 1 | 13.4 | 6 |
| Doughnut, cake-type | 1 oz | 150 | 0 | 12.2 | 6 |

*Source:* Bowes & Church's *Food Values of Portions Commonly Used*, 17th ed., Lippincott, 1998.

products daily. And while not all of these should come to you as a slice of bread, it still leaves a lot of room each day for enjoying the heart-warming goodness of bread and bread products. A serving of bread is one slice, about one ounce or 28 grams. Be aware that when slicing your own from a freshly baked loaf you're likely to serve up a hearty slice that may equal two or even three servings. A bagel, average frozen variety, equals two bread servings, while the king-sized variety may equal four.

Bread-like goodies including scones and muffins most often have added sugar and fat. If you are looking for whole grain, low-fat goodness, be careful when shopping amongst these treats. Many of these baked goods come with unwanted fat, anywhere from one to five teaspoons in a muffin, scone, or croissant. A bran muffin, for example, while a good source of fiber may have over 15 grams of fat in one muffin—that's 135 fat calories! If you can purchase fat-free versions, by all means do. (Check out the "By the Slice" chart for more on these baked goods.) Remember your heart loves bread, not fat.

Tops on my list of favorite foods is fresh baked whole-grain bread slathered with berry fruit spread. What's your favorite way to eat bread? How about a hearty slice to mop spaghetti sauce off your plate, or toasted sourdough bread with a sprinkle of grated Parmesan cheese, fresh basil, and a tomato slice? Stuffed with your favorite sandwich filling or crumbled into a bowl of steamy hot, vegetable soup? Any way you slice it, bread is good, heart-healthy food.

# Breakfast Cereals

Ready-to-eat breakfast cereals are at the top of my list for one of this century's greatest food inventions—boxed wonders. For the most part, breakfast cereals are low in fat, packed with carbo-hydrates, and fortified with an array of vitamins and minerals good for everyday nutrition and good for your heart. Depending on your cereal selection, many are great sources of cholesterol-busting fiber. In fact, studies show that breakfast cereal eaters have lower blood cholesterol levels than non-cereal eaters and breakfast skippers. So if you don't already make cereal a part of your daily menu, your heart wants you to get started as soon as possible.

Ready-to-eat breakfast cereals get their heart-healthy kick from fiber. There are mountains of evidence that cereal fiber cuts the risk of heart disease.

As you know, fiber comes in two types:

- Insoluble fiber that helps relieve constipation, and
- Soluble fiber that helps trap cholesterol in the intestinal tract, preventing it from getting into your circulation.

For years, scientists have studied the cholesterol lowering powers of soluble fiber found in oats, beans, and fruits. Oat-based cereals work wonders on lowering blood cholesterol, especially in people with mild to moderately elevated cholesterol levels (check out page 189 for more on oats).

Another source of soluble fiber found in some cereal is *psyllium,* the husk from the seed of the psyllium plant, found in breakfast cereals such as Kellogg's All-Bran Buds®. When consumed daily, psyllium fiber has been shown to significantly lower blood cholesterol levels.

Very specific research shows that cereal fiber, which is a combination of some soluble, but mostly insoluble fiber, helps fight off heart disease and will even lower high blood pressure. In fact, a recent study tracked the cereal fiber intake of over 43,000 men who were participants in the Health Professionals Follow-up Study. Over a six-year period, the researchers found that those men who had the greatest fiber intake, no matter what their fat intake was, had about two-thirds the risk of suffering from a heart attack compared to men with the lowest fiber intake. The research team felt the evidence was compelling enough to recommend at least a 10-gram per day fiber increase to have a significant effect on heart-disease risk. That's a couple of bowls of whole-grain breakfast cereal.

## Cholesterol-Busting Fiber in a Box

Soluble fiber in some of your favorite oat cereals.

| Cereal | Serving Size | Calories | Total Fiber (gm) | Soluble Fiber (gm) |
|---|---|---|---|---|
| Quaker Oat Bran | 1 1/4 cup | 210 | 6 | 3 |
| Quaker Oatmeal Squares | 1 cup | 220 | 4 | 2 |
| Quaker 100% Natural Low-fat Granola | 1/2 cup | 160 | 2.5 | 1 |

*Source:* Manufacturers' Food Labels

Now we are sure that eating breakfast cereal contributes to lower blood pressure levels. A recent study with children showed that those who took in more fiber, specifically from cereals, had lower blood pressure readings. The fiber in cereal also helps reduce appetite, great news for dieters. Several studies show high-fiber cereal eaters feel full longer, and as a result, eat less at a buffet lunch than those eating a low-fiber cereal.

There is even more good news about the virtues of breakfast cereal. When comparing dietary habits of people who ate cereal for breakfast, traditional eggs and bacon, or skipped breakfast altogether, the cereal eaters came out on top: They had lower blood cholesterol levels and took in less dietary fat for the day, even compared to breakfast skippers who weren't eating a morning meal. Take a look at the cereal charts for your favorite cereals and their fiber content.

**THINGS TO KNOW WHEN CHOOSING A BREAKFAST CEREAL:** Some people avoid cereals thinking their sugar and sodium content may spell trouble. Fear not: When kept at moderate levels, these ingredients won't threaten your heart health.

**Sugar:** Most cereals are made with added sugar. In fact some of the "kiddy" cereals, as well as some adult cereals, are over half

## Bran News

Fiber content of a few ready-to-eat cereals.

| Cereal | Serving Size | Calories | Total Fiber (gm) | Insoluble Fiber (gm) |
|--------|--------------|----------|------------------|----------------------|
| General Mills Fiber One | 1/2 cup | 60 | 13 | 9 |
| Kellogg's All Bran | 1/2 cup | 80 | 10 | 9 |
| Post Shredded Wheat Spoon Size | 1 cup | 170 | 5 | 5 |
| Quaker Corn Bran | 3/4 cup | 90 | 5 | 4 |
| General Mills Wheat Chex | 1 cup | 180 | 5 | 4 |
| General Mills Cheerios | 1 cup | 110 | 3 | 2 |

*Source:* Manufacturers' Food Labels

added sugar. Check out the Nutrition Facts label for sugar on your favorite brand of cereal. Know that every four grams equals one teaspoon of sugar. Some cereals come with a staggering 20 grams or five teaspoons of sugar in a modest three-quarter cup serving! Could you picture yourself spooning that many teaspoons of sugar on a bowl of cereal?

The sugar in cereal, however, does not pose a direct risk for heart disease. Instead, eating a diet high in sugar means there is a good chance you are replacing heart-healthy fruits and vegetables with sugar calories and not getting the fiber from those sources. Consider though, that not much of our daily sugar intake comes from breakfast cereals in the first place. Sodas, candy, cookies, and other foods win that prize. So go ahead, eat breakfast cereals. And if you favor the sugary type, try to mix them in your bowl with a high fiber cereal such as All Bran.

**Sodium:** Since breakfast cereals are a processed food, sodium is typically added. Most cereals have from 150 to 250 milligrams per serving. But some popular brands have over 300

## Adding Milk

How the different milks stack up on your bowl of cereal.

| Milk | Calories | Percent of Calories from Fat | Cholesterol (mg) | Calcium (mg) |
|------|----------|------------------------------|------------------|--------------|
| Whole | 160 | 44% | 35 | 300 |
| Reduced-Fat (2%) | 140 | 32% | 25 | 340 |
| Low-Fat (1%) | 130 | 15% | 15 | 400 |
| Fat-Free (skim) | 90 | 0% | <5 | 300 |
| Soy Milk | 130 | 28% | 0 | 300 |
| Soy Milk (1%) | 100 | 18% | 0 | 20 |
| Soy Milk (nonfat) | 80 | 0% | 0 | 200 |
| Lactose-free (low-fat) | 130 | 35% | 20 | 300 |
| Lactose-free (fat-free) | 90 | 0% | <5 | 300 |
| Buttermilk (1.5%) | 120 | 29% | 15 | 300 |
| Goat Milk | 140 | 43% | 25 | 300 |

*Source:* Manufacturers' Food Labels

milligrams of sodium. As you know, fretting about sodium won't lower your blood pressure; and cereal is far from a high sodium food. So eat breakfast cereal. This is a great food that easily fits in your Simple Six Eating Plan. A bowl of cereal topped with milk is loaded with plenty of nutrients that do more good than bad in combating high blood pressure. See the "Adding Milk" chart for more on cereal toppers.

# Broccoli

A vegetable for all seasons, broccoli is readily available year round in your supermarket's produce section or the freezer aisle. This deep green vegetable, part of the cruciferous family with the likes of Brussels sprouts and cauliflower, comes packed with plenty of heart-smart nutrients. A one-cup serving of cooked broccoli provides a whopping 200 percent of your vitamin C needs and 90 percent of your vitamin A needs as beta carotene. In addition to a generous portion of fiber and a hefty dose of potassium to fight off high blood pressure, broccoli is loaded with other life prolonging ingredients. Frozen broccoli is actually richer in beta carotene than fresh since more of the buds or florets are packaged in the frozen version.

The powerhouses in broccoli, vitamin C and beta carotene, are two of the best known antioxidants that protect all parts of your body from oxidation. As we know from Chapter Two, when LDLs become oxidized or damaged they trigger the heart disease process. Vitamin C and beta carotene, along with vitamin E, keep LDLs from going on their blood vessel ripping rampage. Without a doubt, people who eat more vegetables such as broccoli and get a good intake of vitamin C definitely have a lower risk of heart disease.

And there's more. Broccoli is also a good source of flavonoids. These substances, also found in tea, onions, and other fruits and vegetables, protect you from heart attack risk. Like the antioxidants, vitamins C and E, flavonoids also act to protect LDLs from becoming artery-damaging grenades. The more flavonoids you take in, the lower your risk for heart disease. There is also some preliminary scientific work showing that when we are put under stress that normally would increase our heart attack risk, flavonoids help reduce this risk by making the blood less likely to cause life-threatening clots.

Purchase fresh or frozen broccoli. When selecting fresh, choose firm dense florets. Fresh broccoli keeps for about five to seven days stored wrapped in your refrigerator. Before cooking, rinse in cold water and cut into pieces that are bigger than bite-size. The smaller the pieces during cooking, the greater the nutrient loss. Microwave or steam broccoli three to five minutes until slightly tender and bright green. Use cooked broccoli florets in omelets or green salads. Also put uncooked broccoli in casseroles, soups, or during the last few minutes of cooking for stews (so as not to make the broccoli too mushy). Broccoli is also a great stir-fry staple. Of course, you can always eat broccoli raw—it's great dipped in a low-fat sour cream and fresh herb mixture. Try my Broccoli Sesame Salad recipe for a refreshing side dish.

### Broccoli-Sesame Salad

1 1/2 cups broccoli florets—about 1 1/2 inches in length

1 tbsp. canola oil

1 tsp. sesame oil

2 tsp. sesame seeds

2 cups mixed greens (arugala, romaine, red leaf lettuce)

1/2 cup thinly sliced cucumber

1/4 cup thinly sliced red onion

2 tbsp. raspberry vinegar

In a nonstick wok, heat the oils and then add the broccoli. Stir-fry for two minutes then turn down heat and cover a few minutes until bright green and slightly tender to the poke of a fork. Add sesame seeds and toss. Set aside to cool (can be refrigerated to cool). In a salad bowl, combine greens, cucumber, and onion slices. Add cooled broccoli and toss with vinegar. Serves four.

## Nutrition Facts

Broccoli-Sesame Salad

Serving Size 1/4 recipe

| Amount per Serving | |
|---|---|
| Calories 72 | 50 Calories from fat |
| | % Daily Value |
| Total Fat 6g | 9% |
| Saturated Fat <1g | 3% |
| Cholesterol 0mg | 0% |
| Sodium 13mg | 1% |
| Total Carbohydrate 5g | 2% |
| Dietary Fiber 2g | 8% |
| Protein 2g | |

| | | |
|---|---|---|
| Vitamin A 14% | • | Vitamin C 66% |
| Calcium 3% | • | Iron 5% |

# Butter

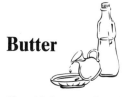

Should I state the obvious? Butter is not exactly a heart-healthy food, but you know that. In fact, you probably think of butter as the opposite—a heart-attack food. And rightly so; after all, butter is loaded with saturated fat. And that is the kind of fat we want to minimize in our diet. But, while butter shouldn't be a dietary staple, there is room for just a bit. Research shows us that opting for stick margarine over butter for slathering on your bread does not have the heart-saving benefit you may have thought. It all boils (or melts) down to the type of saturated fat found in butter and what impact this has on blood cholesterol levels.

Butter stats certainly aren't pretty: One tablespoon has 108 calories, with all of them coming from fat and 33 milligrams of cholesterol to boot. And over half the fat in butter is saturated, the solid, artery-clogging fat you are advised to keep at a minimum in your diet. However, not all saturated fats are created equal. A saturated fat that is common in butter is called *stearic acid.* This saturated fat has been shown not to raise blood cholesterol levels the same way other common saturated fats do. (Stearic acid is also found in chocolate and beef.)

While this news does not mean you can butter up everything from bread to vegetables, it is nice to know that you don't have to avoid butter like the plague. Many people opt for margarine as a spread alternative in hopes of avoiding mischief with blood cholesterol levels. But margarine does not appear to be the "better" spread when it comes to heart health. Margarine, particularly the stick type, has a type of fat called *trans* fat which raises blood cholesterol levels and appears to be equally as damaging to the heart or maybe more so than saturated fats.

Scientists from the Netherlands reviewed 20 different research studies that examined the effect of using butter or margarine on blood cholesterol levels. They concluded that butter was no better, or no worse, than stick margarine when in came to heart-disease risk. This means that saving on butter's saturated fat by substituting it with margarine's *trans* fats is a bust.

Overall, you're better off cutting back on total fat intake in the diet. The Netherlands researchers also concluded that soft-type "spreadable" margarines (often sold in tubs) actually do cut risk for heart disease when used in place of butter. I suggest you use soft margarine which is lower in *trans* fats, or even diet margarines where real butter taste won't be missed. Occasionally, and on occasion, using butter is certainly okay. (I have more to say on how to choose margarines, so check out Margarine on page 175 for what's best to use.)

Here are some heart-healthy tips on how butter can fit into your diet.

## Butter Stats

Check out how your favorite spread compares.

| Butter | Calories | Fat grams (gm) | Satu-rated (gm) | Trans (gm) | Chol-esterol (mg) | Sodium (mg) |
|---|---|---|---|---|---|---|
| Butter, unsalted | 100 | 11 | 7 | 0 | 30 | 0 |
| Butter, sweet | 100 | 11 | 7 | 0 | 30 | 90 |
| Whipped butter | 60 | 7 | 5 | 0 | 20 | 55 |
| Reduced-fat butter | 50 | 6 | 4 | 0 | 20 | 70 |
| Margarine, stick | 90 | 10 | 1.5 | 2 | 0 | 100 |
| Margarine, tub | 100 | 11 | 1 | 0 | 0 | 110 |
| Low-fat Margarine | 50 | 6 | 1 | 0 | 0 | 75 |
| Squeeze | 80 | 9 | 1.5 | 1 | 0 | 110 |
| Fat-free | 5 | 0 | 0 | 0 | 0 | 130 |

*Source:* Manufacturers' Food Labels

- Evaluate your use of added fat such as salad dressings, butter, or margarine spread on breads, bagels, cooked pasta, or vegetables.
- Also, add up any oil you use in cooking.
- Limit yourself to no more than five teaspoons of added fat per day. (Know that one teaspoon of butter has five grams of fat.)
- Combine this with fat you eat daily from processed and other foods, and then total your fat intake for the day. It shouldn't exceed 13 teaspoons or 65 grams on average. (Go back and check out your Simple Six Eating Plan for your specific fat budget—see Chapter Two.)
- If your saturated fat intake from other foods is low, you can fit in one or two teaspoons of butter daily.
- Small amounts of butter go a long way when it comes to taste. Scratch just a tad across a warm toasted bagel or muffin.
- Keep butter soft by bringing to room temperature before use. Soft butter spreads more thinly so you get away with using less.
- When following a recipe that calls for butter, you can save some fat by cutting back on total use. Also, as a way to keep the butter taste and not all the saturated fat, substitute in some soft margarine.

# Cabbage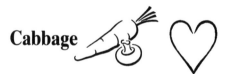

It's not exactly everyone's favorite vegetable, but if eating away heart disease and high blood pressure is your goal, take another look at cabbage. This lowly vegetable comes packed with a host of nutrients that fend off disease. But most of us think of cabbage as a smelly, not-so-chic vegetable. Perhaps cabbage's bad image got started during World War II when it became a staple in Europe during the lean war years. Since citrus fruits were scarce, this vegetable became the major source of vitamin C for war-torn England. As a result, some people regard cabbage as a sign of tough times.

One cup of shredded, raw cabbage gives you almost 70 percent of your vitamin C needs and a good dose of potassium to help fight high blood pressure. Green cabbage, more so than red, supplies about 10 percent of folate needs. This B vitamin helps fight heart disease by clearing artery-damaging homocysteine from the circulation. And besides all this, cabbage comes equipped with cholesterol-clearing fiber and only 20 calories per serving.

The only disadvantage of cabbage (and maybe a reason you have stayed away from it in the past) is its bad, sulfur-like smell when it's cooked. In fact, the more you cook cabbage, the more it stinks. Fresh cabbage tastes great raw mixed into green salads or on its own as coleslaw (you can purchase ready-made reduced-fat or nonfat coleslaw dressings). Flash cook cabbage by quickly stir-frying or lightly steaming. This keeps odors down and nutrients in. Fresh cabbage is also a great keeper—stored in a tightly wrapped plastic bag in your refrigerator it will stay fresh for weeks. Try my heart-smart, stir-fried Chinese-style burritos.

### *Stir-Fry Cabbage and Tofu Mu-Shu Style*

2 cups chopped green cabbage

1/2 cup Chinese cabbage, shredded

1/2 cup scallions, chopped

1 cup firm tofu, cut in small cubes (can substitute scrambled eggs or diced chicken)

1/3 cup bottled stir-fry sauce

4 Chinese-style pancakes/tortillas/wraps

2 tbsp. plum sauce

In a bowl, toss tofu with sauce and put aside. In a nonstick wok (or use small amount of canola oil), stir-fry cabbage and scallions quickly and remove. Stir-fry tofu until heated through and then add vegetables. Serve on heated tortillas with plum sauce. Serves four.

**Nutrition Facts**

Stir-Fry Cabbage and Tofu Mu-Shu Style
Serving Size 1/4 recipe

| Amount per Serving | |
| --- | --- |
| Calories 204 | 50 Calories from fat |

| | % Daily Value |
| --- | --- |
| Total Fat 5g | 8% |
| Saturated Fat <1g | 4% |
| Cholesterol 0mg | 0% |
| Sodium 840mg | 35% |
| Total Carbohydrate 32g | 11% |
| Dietary Fiber 3g | 12% |
| Protein 10g | |

| | | |
| --- | --- | --- |
| Vitamin A 3% | • | Vitamin C 36% |
| Calcium 11% | • | Iron 24% |
| Folate 15% | • | Vitamin E 32% |

# Canola Oil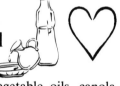

Among the vegetable oils, canola oil stands out as the heart-healthy choice. This all-purpose cooking and eating oil has the lowest level of artery-clogging saturated fat and is rich in monoun-saturated fats, the good guys that help lower blood cholesterol levels. Studies show that diets rich in monounsatured fats, such as canola or olive oil, help lower heart-disease risk. But it's olive oil, not canola, that people typically choose when thinking about their hearts. All things considered though, canola is just as good as olive oil, and in some ways, it's better.

For starters, when it comes to heart health, canola oil is just as effective as olive oil in lowering blood cholesterol levels. Research from the University of Uppsala in Sweden demonstrated that when canola oil replaced saturated fats in the diets' of participants, cholesterol levels dropped the same amount as with olive oil. And just like olive oil, canola didn't tamper with HDL levels.

Canola oil might have an edge on olive oil's fat stats. In each tablespoon, both oils have the same number of calories and grams of fat—124 and 14; but canola is lower in saturated fat: one gram versus two in olive oil. And more good news, canola oil has a small

### Fat Chance

Compare canola oil with your favorite cooking fat for heart-healthy monounsaturated fats.

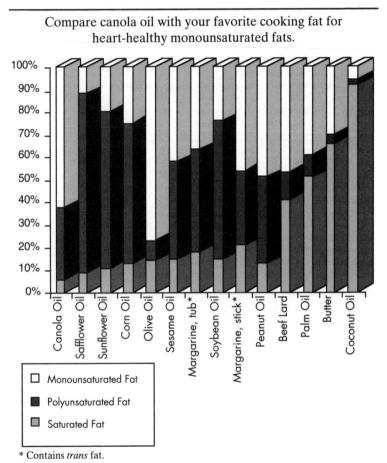

☐ Monounsaturated Fat

■ Polyunsaturated Fat

▨ Saturated Fat

* Contains *trans* fat.

amount of omega-3 fats, the same type found in fish. The amazing power of omega-3 has been shown throughout the scientific community to help reduce heart-disease risk and lower blood pressure. Check out the "Fat Chance" chart for more information.

But don't go deep frying your taters in canola oil. As always, a diet with less than 30 percent fat calories is recommended. Since many of us consume more fat than is recommended, cut back on added fat and switch to canola oil in place of saturated fats such as stick margarine, vegetable shortening, or butter. Replacing some polyunsaturated fats—corn, sunflower, and safflower oils—with canola is also a good idea. Ideally, you want your diet to have more monounsaturated than saturated or polyunsaturated fats.

Unlike olive oil, canola doesn't come in "virgin" and "extra virgin" varieties, making your selection process simpler. Canola oil is virtually tasteless and less expensive than olive. So when you're not after that Italian flare, use canola oil.

In an effort to use less fat when cooking, try an oil pump spray available at kitchen stores and department stores. This simple device sprays oil in a fine mist on the cooking surface. This way you can avoid pouring unnecessary oil into a skillet for a stir-fry—just spray the surface and you're ready to sauté.

# Cantaloupe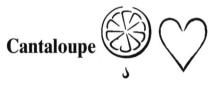

Juicy and sweet, cantaloupe is one of summer's finest gems. This fruit's claim to fame when it comes to heart health is what I call a "triple power play." Cantaloupe is packed with three no-nonsense heart disease and high blood pressure fighting nutrients: vitamin C, beta carotene, and potassium.

One cup of fresh cantaloupe pieces supplies over 100 percent of vitamin C needs along with over 60 percent of the beta carotene needs recommended for heart health. This duo helps to keep LDLs from becoming oxidized and damaging to artery walls. As researchers learn more about what triggers artery damage and cholesterol buildup in the first place, they are finding out that vitamin C and beta carotene play a major role as part of a much larger nutrition-based repair team that keeps heart disease at bay.

Cantaloupe is also brimming with potassium. When it comes to this mineral, cantaloupe outshines even bananas. Recent research shows that this mineral puts a powerful damper on high blood pressure. A study from Harvard School of Public Health showed that when women boosted their potassium intake from marginal levels, blood pressure dropped dramatically. This mineral works on high blood pressure through controlling fluid balance in the circulation, countering the action of sodium.

The best time for cantaloupe is during the dog days of summer when most other melons are in season. At other times, you can purchase imported melons for a higher price, or buy frozen cantaloupe sold packaged into bite-size pieces. When buying fresh, look for firm, ripe melons that have a sweet smell. Avoid overly ripe cantaloupe by checking the end for a mushy feel. Chill your cantaloupe before serving. Try melon pieces in smoothies, in fruit salads, or as a colorfully sweet addition to green salads. Surprisingly, cantaloupe makes a great base for a fruit salsa—see my recipe on page 239. My favorite way to eat cantaloupe, and perhaps the simplest—slice a chilled melon into quarters, remove the seeds, and sprinkle each slice with a touch of fresh lemon juice. Invite three friends over and enjoy!

# Carrots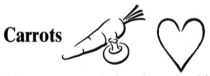

Almost everyone's favorite vegetable is the carrot, and for good reason. Carrot munching is an easy way to protect your heart. This vegetable's name and color reflects its best known nutrient—it's packed with beta carotene, which studies show may help reduce heart-disease risk. One medium carrot has over 200 percent of your vitamin A needs as beta carotene. Beta carotene acts as a powerful antioxidant that helps protect those bad carriers of cholesterol, LDLs, from becoming oxidized. When in the oxidized state, LDLs tear up artery walls, leading to the first stages of heart disease.

In a study from Southwestern Medical Center in Dallas, researchers discovered that when beta carotene intake of participants was increased, their LDLs were less susceptible to becoming oxidized or damaged. This means that in the body, these "softer, gentler" LDLs will not cause the damage to artery walls that results in cholesterol buildup and clogged vessels.

What makes carrots such a great heart protector is that it's so easy to get plenty of beta carotene from eating just one carrot. And since carrots are such a versatile veggie, you can easily fit these orange gems into your daily menu. Eat carrot sticks raw as a quick snack or mobile munchy while working or driving. The popular baby carrots sold ready-to-eat in resealable bags have just as much beta carotene as the standard long variety. You can also shred raw carrots and toss them into green salads, use in sandwiches, or blend into smoothies. Or try my Carrot-Walnut-Raisin Salad for a blast of beta carotene.

Cooked carrots retain much of their beta carotene. Steam or microwave carrots, top with fresh herbs, and use as a side dish. Or add sliced carrots to stir-frys, stews, or soups. Carrots boiled with potatoes in a vegetable broth along with some seasonings blend nicely into a "cream" of carrot soup. Let me tell you a cooking secret using carrots: To take the acidic bite out of spaghetti sauce, add fresh minced carrots (food-processor style) to the sauce an hour before serving. Now you have a mellow, smooth, heart-healthy sauce for pasta, lasagna, or pizza. And there is always room for carrot cake or carrot muffins made with applesauce in place of all or some of the oil called for in the recipe (see recipe starting on page 225).

### *Carrot-Walnut-Raisin Salad*

2 cups shredded carrots (use food processor or grater)

1/4 cup chopped walnuts

1/2 cup raisins

1/2 cup nonfat vanilla yogurt

1/4 cup crushed pineapple (optional)

Mix all ingredients in a bowl. Chill at least 30 minutes before serving. Makes four servings.

| **Nutrition Facts** Carrot-Walnut-Raisin Salad Serving Size 1/4 recipe | |
|---|---|
| Amount per Serving | |
| Calories 158 | 42 Calories from fat |
| | % Daily Value |
| Total Fat 5g | 7% |
| Saturated Fat <1g | 2% |
| Cholesterol 0mg | 0% |
| Sodium 44mg | 2% |
| Total Carbohydrate 27g | 9% |
| Dietary Fiber 3g | 14% |
| Protein 5g | |
| Vitamin A 180% • Vitamin C 13% Calcium 10% • Iron 6% | |

# Cauliflower

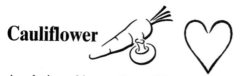

A relative of broccoli, cauliflower comes brimming with nutrients for a healthier heart. One cup of raw cauliflower, or a half cup cooked has a mere 25 calories and about three grams of fiber. This vegetable also has an array of heart-smart nutrients:

- over 100 percent of vitamin C needs,
- almost 20 percent of your folate requirement, and
- at least 10 percent of vitamin $B_6$ and potassium needs.

These handful of nutrients go to work for you protecting your heart. Folate and vitamin $B_6$, for example, both play a role in the breakdown of the blood factor called *homocysteine* that is known to cause artery damage.

Even though related to broccoli, cauliflower lacks the green chlorophyll that gives broccoli a tarter taste. As a result, cauliflower has a more bland taste but this works well in dishes as it doesn't overpower the flavor of other ingredients. Use cauliflower raw in bite-size pieces in salads or for dipping in Indian bean dip called *hummus.* Also use cauliflower in stir-fry or soup; or steam and toss with freshly grated Parmesan cheese and black pepper and use as a side dish to accompany fish, chicken, or pasta. Cauliflower keeps a good one to two weeks in the refrigerator and can also be purchased frozen in ready-to-use pieces.

### *Cauliflower and Potato Curry*

1 large white onion, chopped

1 tsp. fresh ginger, finely chopped

1 tsp. chopped garlic

2 cloves

1 cinnamon stick or bark

1 tsp. turmeric

5 potatoes, cubed (leave skin)

5 tomatoes, chopped

1 head of cauliflower, chopped into 2-inch pieces

3 tbsp. olive oil

In a large skillet, heat oil and add onions, ginger, garlic, cloves, and cinnamon. Sauté until onion is soft. Add potatoes, tomatoes, and one cup of water. Cover and cook over medium heat until potatoes are half-way cooked (about 10 minutes). Then add cauliflower and cook another 10 to 15 minutes or until cauliflower is tender. Garnish with fresh chopped corriander and serve with rice. Makes six servings.

| **Nutrition Facts** | |
| --- | --- |
| Cauliflower and Potato Curry | |
| Serving Size 1/6 recipe | |
| Amount per Serving | |
| Calories 123 | 72 Calories from fat |
| | % Daily Value |
| Total Fat 7g | 11% |
|    Saturated Fat 1g | 5% |
| Cholesterol 0mg | 0% |
| Sodium 22mg | 1% |
| Total Carbohydrate 14g | 5% |
|    Dietary Fiber 4g | 16% |
| Protein 3g | |
| Vitamin A 7% • Vitamin C 97% | |
| Calcium 4% • Iron 15% | |
| Folate 13% • Vitamin B$_6$ 14% | |

# Celery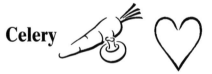

A rather unsuspecting vegetable, celery packs a punch when it comes to fighting high blood pressure. Most are surprised when checking out celery's nutritional profile. One stalk, about 8 inches long, has 40 calories and just over 120 milligrams of potassium—5 percent of your minimum needs. But there's more. Celery packs an array of phytochemicals; one in particular helps ward off high blood pressure.

Celery contains 3-n-butyl phthalide, a mouthful to say, but a phytochemical that's good for your heart. In a laboratory study using animals, blood pressure dropped over 10 percent following treatment with 3-n-butyl phthalide. Researchers theorize this phytochemical affects the levels of stress hormones in the body that may trigger high blood pressure in some people.

Even though munching on celery shouldn't replace blood pressure medication, including a stalk or two in your daily fare adds to the food arsenal against the bad guys. Try celery in stir-fry dishes or add to ready-made soups (a little extra heating time is needed to cook the celery). Add raw celery to salads or mix into tuna salad (low-fat or nonfat mayo, please) for a refreshing crunch. And of course, gnawing on raw celery sticks makes a great anytime snack. When shopping, make sure to select firm celery stalks that are not wilted or yellowed. Try this delicious "Cream" of Celery Soup recipe for a warming heart-healthy meal.

## *"Cream" of Celery Soup*

1 onion, chopped

2 cans low-sodium vegetable broth

ground pepper to taste

1/2 tsp. dill

2 large potatoes, sliced

2 cloves of garlic, crushed

7 stalks of celery, chopped

red pepper flakes to taste (optional)

In a soup pot, sauté the onions and garlic in 1 tablespoon olive oil until slightly limp. Add the celery and sauté a few more minutes. Add the potato slices, pour in the vegetable broth and blend in seasonings. Bring mixture to a boil, then reduce heat and simmer for 30 minutes or until vegetables are soft. With a hand mixer or a blender, "cream" the soup mixture until all ingredients are well blended. Serves four to six.

| Nutrition Facts | |
| --- | --- |
| "Cream" of Celery Soup | |
| Serving Size 1 cup | |
| Amount per Serving | |
| Calories 100        9 Calories from fat | |
| | % Daily Value |
| Total Fat 1g | <1% |
| Saturated Fat 0g | 0% |
| Cholesterol 0mg | 0% |
| Sodium 200mg | 8% |
| Total Carbohydrate 22g | 7% |
| Dietary Fiber 2.5g | 10% |
| Protein 4g        8% | |
| Vitamin A 1%    •  Vitamin C 25% | |
| Calcium 4%      •  Iron 10% | |

# Cheese

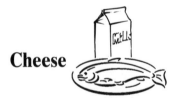

What I call an "Old World" food, cheese has been around for thousands of years. Some think cheese has no place in a heart-healthy diet because of its high fat content. I am happy to report to you that leading researchers conclude there is no convincing evidence that links cheese consumption to heart disease. In fact, cheese makes a regular appearance in "Mediterranean" diets, noted for their ability to reduce heart-disease risk. Bottom line for cheese lovers: Eating cheese in modest amounts presents no harm to your heart.

A quick look at cheese's profile initially may make your heart skip a beat. On average an ounce of hard cheese such as cheddar or Swiss has about 110 calories and 9 grams of fat, or about 70 percent or so of the calories from fat. And most of this fat—roughly 60 percent—is saturated, not so great news for arteries. Most cheeses also have about 20-plus milligrams of cholesterol, slightly less than 10 percent of your daily budget. Soft cheeses, such as goat and ricotta cheeses, often are lower in fat content but there are big exceptions. Cream cheese, for example, has more fat per ounce than cheddar.

Cheeses also come packed with a hefty dose of sodium. Most cheeses have about 150 to over 200 milligrams per serving. And processed cheeses have even more—400 milligrams in a serving of processed American cheese slices.

But cheese certainly has some attributes worth mentioning that may help explain why heart disease rates are lower among people who include modest amounts of cheese in their diets. Cheese is a great source of calcium. This mineral not only builds strong bones, but studies show that people who consume adequate calcium have an easier time keeping blood pressure levels in check. A one-ounce serving of most cheese contains about 20 percent of the Daily Value for calcium.

### Say Yes to Cheese?

So knowing all this grim news about the fat and sodium in cheese, why isn't it on the "most unwanted" list for foods against healthy hearts? According to research from the Mediterranean regions of Europe, low heart disease rates are attributable to certain dietary habits—daily intake of fresh fruits, vegetables, olive oil, and modest amounts of cheese and yogurt. A very "Mediterranean" meal, for example, is pasta topped lightly with grated full-fat but flavorful hard cheese, a side dish of vegetables and fruit for dessert.

The key in using cheese as part of your Simple Six Eating Plan is the "modest" amount. One to two ounces used sparingly is the way to incorporate cheese into your diet. Cheeses add flavor, even tang to a dish. But slathering a bagel with cream cheese, or drowning nachos with melted cheese adds more fat and so-dium than you bargained for. Try using small amounts of strong flavored cheeses such as Parmesan or blue cheese grated or crumbled over a green salad. This way you can appreciate the

## Say Cheese

How does your favorite cheese fare when it comes to fat and saturated fat?

| Cheese (1 oz.) | Calories | Fat (gm) | Saturated Fat (gm) | Sodium (mg) |
|---|---|---|---|---|
| American (1 slice) | 60 | 4 | 3 | 300 |
| Blue Cheese | 110 | 9 | 6 | 400 |
| Cheddar | 110 | 9 | 5 | 180 |
| Cream Cheese | 100 | 10 | 7 | 100 |
| Goat | 50 | 4 | 2.5 | 120 |
| Gouda | 100 | 8 | 6 | 210 |
| Monterey Jack | 100 | 8 | 5 | 170 |
| Mozzarella | 80 | 5 | 3 | 170 |
| Parmesan | 25 | 1.5 | 1 | 90 |
| Provolone | 150 | 11 | 8 | 370 |
| Ricotta | 100 | 6 | 4 | 80 |
| Swiss | 100 | 8 | 5 | 10 |
| Cheese Whiz | 100 | 8 | 4 | 470 |

*Source:* Manufacturers' Food Labels

tangy flavor without piling on calories and fat. Use cheese as a garnish atop casseroles and entrées such as chicken or fish.

### Lower Fat Options

Over the past several years, reduced-fat and nonfat cheeses have been making their appearance alongside full-fat versions. These lower fat varieties can save you anywhere from 30 to 100 percent of the fat calories. Many come with a notable level of sodium—100 to 300 milligrams (unless they are marked low-sodium). Fat-reduced cheeses are also a good source of calcium and protein.

# Cheese Line-Up

Check out the fat savings with reduced fat and fat-free options.

| Fat-Free and Low-Fat | Calories | Fat (gm) | Saturated (gm) | Sodium (mg) |
|---|---|---|---|---|
| Low-Fat Mozzarella (1 oz.) | 70 | 3 | 2 | 180 |
| Nonfat Mozzarella (1/4 cup) | 45 | 0 | 0 | 200 |
| Reduced-Fat Cheddar (1 oz.) | 90 | 6 | 4 | 240 |
| Nonfat Cheddar (1/4 cup) | 45 | 0 | 0 | 200 |
| Reduced-Fat Swiss (1 slice) | 80 | 4 | 2.5 | 50 |
| Fat-Free Swiss | 45 | 0 | 0 | 290 |
| Low-Fat Cream Cheese (2 tbsp.) | 70 | 5 | 3.5 | 160 |
| Nonfat Cream Cheese (2 tbsp.) | 30 | 0 | 0 | 200 |
| Low-Fat Ricotta (1/4 cup) | 70 | 3 | 1.5 | 45 |
| Fat-Free Ricotta (1/4 cup) | 50 | 0 | 0 | 150 |
| Reduced-Fat Monterey Jack (1 oz.) | 80 | 6 | 4 | 240 |
| American | 60 | 4 | 3 | 300 |
| Low-Fat American | 60 | 3 | 2 | 290 |
| Fat-Free American | 30 | 0 | 0 | 280 |

*Source:* Manufacturers' Food Labels

## Look Before You Cheese

Compare the fat savings when you select a low-fat cheese instead of its full-fat counterpart.

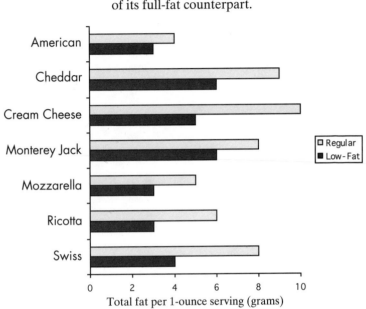

Total fat per 1-ounce serving (grams)

While brands vary, lower-fat cheeses taste pretty good. Their melting consistency, however, is less than desirable so many of these cheeses are best used in sandwiches, on salads, and in burritos or tacos. Making a cheese sauce may be tricky as some nonfat cheeses get rubbery when melted. Compare fat and calorie savings with reduced-fat and nonfat cheeses in the chart on the previous page.

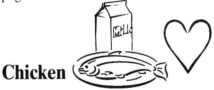

# Chicken

Chicken makes a great fit in your Simple Six Eating Plan. A three-ounce serving of white chicken meat has just three grams of fat—about 19 percent of the total calories—with a third of it coming from heart-healthy monounsaturated fat. To boot, chicken is a great source of vitamin $B_6$ that helps lower homocysteine levels (an artery-damaging substance in the blood), and a fabulous source of protein—a staggering 50 percent of the Daily Value in one three-ounce serving.

According to several studies, chicken as part of a low-fat diet aimed at lowering blood cholesterol levels works wonders. In a recent study, a group of people ate chicken daily or every other day in moderate amounts (three ounces as a serving). Blood cholesterol levels fell as expected with a diet low in fatty foods. Numerous studies show that chicken fits in well with diets designed to lower high blood pressure. In the now famous "DASH" study, blood pressure dropped in participants who ate a low-fat diet packed with fruits and vegetables which included moderate amounts of chicken (see page 296 for more on the DASH diet).

Some people skip chicken, as well as other meats, for fear of the cholesterol in poultry and other meats. Your daily cholesterol tally should be kept below 300 milligrams. A serving of chicken easily fits, as the cholesterol content is about 70 to 80 milligrams per serving, comparable to the same amount of beef. Dietary intake of cholesterol is not as threatening to your circulating levels of cholesterol as once thought. Also, many other items in the diet such as total fat and saturated fat intake play a much larger role in tampering with your blood cholesterol levels and your risk for heart disease.

### Chicken Fixins'

Select either frozen or fresh chicken and use within three days if stored in the refrigerator. Chicken keeps well frozen for about six months. Bake, microwave, or grill chicken. While cooked chicken skin may taste great, peel it off before eating to save on fat. You may even take the skin off before cooking, but this does not save much in the way of fat and the skin does help keep the meat moist during baking. (Just remember to take the skin off before eating.) Frying chicken in oil is a no-no as this adds a significant amount of

## Fixin' Chicken

See for yourself how frying chicken adds unwanted fat calories.

| Chicken, 3 oz. Serving Size | Calories | Fat (grams) | Percent Calories from Fat |
|---|---|---|---|
| *Baked* | | | |
| breast, skinless | 142 | 3.1 | 20% |
| thigh, skinless | 163 | 8.6 | 47% |
| drumstick, skinless | 152 | 5 | 29% |
| *Fried* | | | |
| breast, with skin | 192 | 7.7 | 36% |
| thigh, with skin | 226 | 13 | 52% |
| wing, with skin | 278 | 16 | 52% |

unwanted fat—even if you removed the fried outer batter and skin layer. (See the "Fixin' Chicken" chart above for more information.) If you like the taste of crispy chicken, try my recipe for Oven "Fried" Chicken. The buttermilk is the secret to its great taste!

## *Oven "Fried" Chicken*

fresh or frozen chicken, half-breasts and thighs, skin removed

1 cup buttermilk

2 cups bread crumbs

1/2 tsp. fresh ground pepper

Prepare baking sheet by lining bottom with aluminum foil. In a sturdy plastic bag, place bread crumbs and pepper. Taking one piece at a time, dip chicken into buttermilk (previously poured into a low bowl) and then place into plastic bag. Secure the bag tightly with your hands and shake to cover chicken piece with bread crumbs. Remove chicken from bag and place on baking sheet. Repeat this for all the pieces of chicken—enough for about 10 pieces of chicken. Bake covered with foil in a 375 degree oven for 45 minutes, then remove the foil covering and bake an additional 15 minutes. Chicken should not appear pink inside and juices should run clear. A serving is three ounces, about 1/2 breast or 1 1/2 thigh pieces.

| **Nutrition Facts** | |
|---|---|
| Oven "Fried" Chicken | |
| Serving Size 3 oz. | |
| Amount per Serving | |
| Calories 227 | 36 Calories from fat |
| | % Daily Value |
| Total Fat 4g | 6% |
| Saturated Fat 1g | 6% |
| Cholesterol 74mg | 25% |
| Sodium 230mg | 10% |
| Total Carbohydrate 16g | 5% |
| Dietary Fiber 1g | 3% |
| Protein 30g | |
| Vitamin A <2% • Vitamin C 0% | |
| Calcium 6% • Iron 10% | |

# Chips

Chips are a favorite snack food for most of us. On average, every man, woman, and child in the U.S. eats a staggering 22 pounds of potato chips, tortilla chips, and the like each year. And considering one ounce, about 15 chips, is a serving, this means we average one serving of chips each day! Chips are loaded with fat and sodium. Each serving packs about 150 calories, 10 grams of fat contributing

## Chip off the Ol' Block

Check the fat content of your favorite chips.

| *Chips*<br>*(1 oz.)* | *Calories* | *Percent*<br>*Calories*<br>*from Fat* | *Sodium*<br>*(mg)* |
|---|---|---|---|
| *Potato Chips* | | | |
| Lay's Classic | 150 | 60 | 180 |
| Baked Lay's | 110 | 13 | 150 |
| Lay's WOW® Fat-Free | 75 | 0 | 180 |
| Ruffles | 160 | 56 | 180 |
| Reduced-Fat Ruffles | 140 | 45 | 130 |
| Ruffles WOW® Fat-Free | 75 | 0 | 190 |
| Pringles Original | 160 | 62 | 170 |
| Pringles Original 1/3 less fat | 140 | 7 | 135 |
| Pringles Fat-Free | 70 | 0 | 160 |
| Guiltless Gourmet<br>Baked not Fried | 110 | 12 | 180 |
| | | | |
| *Tortilla/Corn Chips* | | | |
| Doritos Cool Ranch | 140 | 43 | 170 |
| Doritos Cool Ranch Reduced-Fat | 130 | 35 | 200 |
| Doritos WOW® Fat-Free | 90 | 10 | 240 |
| Tostitos White Corn<br>Restaurant Style | 130 | 42 | 80 |
| Baked Tostitos Low-Fat Unsalted | 110 | 8 | 0 |
| Padrino's Nacho Cheese | 130 | 55 | 210 |
| Padrino's Nacho Cheese<br>Reduced-Fat | 120 | 30 | 210 |
| Guiltless Gourmet Original<br>Baked not Fried | 110 | 8 | 160 |
| Fritos Original | 180 | 50 | 160 |

*Source:* Manufacturers' Food Labels

60 percent of the calories, and 150 to 200 milligrams of sodium. And who can eat just one? Most people devour several servings of chips at a time, making them even more of a diet disaster.

But don't despair, you can have your chips and eat them too. A little chip-eating savvy can keep you on track. For starters, many major brands have reduced-fat or even fat-free versions of chips that taste great. This option certainly helps save on fat and calories, but the sodium content is still high. And keep in mind that reduced-fat chips only have a third less fat than the originals, 6.7 grams versus 10 grams, which adds up quickly. So gobbling down two servings of reduced-fat chips instead of one of the regular version ends up being worse all the way around. Check the "Chip off the Ol' Block" chart for comparisons on regular and lower-fat chip choices.

Fat-free chips offer the chip lover a guiltless alternative, as long as some restraint is used. Many of the fat-free versions are baked chips, giving them a much different texture and flavor compared to the real thing. This difference in taste alone may keep you from eating more than just one. But the recently introduced chips made with the fat substitute, Olestra, with the trade name *Olean*, tastes like the real thing. These chips, sold under the brand name of Wow®, have half the calories of regular chips and are fat free. And according to consumer taste tests and astronomical sales—$58 million in its first eight weeks on the market—Wow® chips taste like the real thing.

## Easy Dipping

| *Best Choices* | *Use Sparingly* |
| --- | --- |
| tomato salsa | sour cream |
| green salsa | cream cheese dip |
| hummus (blended chickpeas) | processed cheese dips |
| fruit salsa | full-fat bean dip |
| reduced-fat bean dip | guacamole made with mayo or |
| guacamole (my recipe on page 63) | sour cream |

Great taste and no fat, however, doesn't give you carte blanche to gobble down multiple servings. Olestra is a fat substitute, to be used as such. Olestra-based chips are not calorie free, and are not free of potential side effects. Chips made with Olestra come with a warning that the product may cause abdominal cramping and loose stools. Also, as Olestra passes through the digestive tract into your stool, it takes along with it crucial fat-soluble vitamins like vitamins A and E. As a result, the Food and Drug Administration requires chip makers to fortify their products with extra vitamins.

Perhaps more crucial is how these fat-free chips help you eat away heart disease. There's no solid evidence that eating chips made with Olestra provides any benefit in lowering blood cholesterol levels and heart-disease risk. And keeping sodium levels in check can be a struggle with multiple servings of Olestra chips (or any chips for that matter).

**Bottom line on chips:** Eat chips, whether fat-free or regular, in modest amounts. Here are more tips on chip eating to keep your heart healthy.

### Chip Tips

- Choose chips that have less than 130 calories per serving, less than three grams of fat and less than 150 milligrams of sodium.
- Flavored chips, such as bar-b-que, nacho cheese, and ranch, have more sodium per serving than regular chips.
- Measure out one serving of chips according to the package label and take note. Are you eating just one serving?
- Read the label for the type of fat used in chip making. Avoid hydrogenated vegetable oils since these contain cholesterol-raising *trans* fats.
- Chic "vegetable chips" made from carrots, beets, or sweet potatoes are just as fatty and salty as regular chips and provide little nutritional advantage.
- Potato chips made with the skin offer no significant advantage over the "skinless" varieties.

- When chip dipping, use fresh tomato and chili salsas or fruit salsas for a dose of great tasting heart-healthy ingredients. Or use slim dips made with fat-free sour cream or yogurt and fresh herbs. Check the "Easy Dipping" chart for more suggestions.

# Chocolate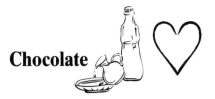

The ancient Aztec civilizations knew a good thing when they tasted it. They actually used cocoa beans as a form of money. And as any good self-respecting chocoholic, I too have bartered with family and friends for a piece of chocolate. But as most people know, including us chocoholics, this delicacy is loaded with fat and calories and hardly can be thought of as a heart-healthy food. But wait . . . (thank goodness) new research shows chocolate contains the same phytochemicals that are found in red wine, which fight against heart disease!

Scientists from the enology (study of wine) department from the University of California at Davis discovered that chocolate contains significant amounts of *phenols,* the same protective agents in red wine. Andrew Waterhouse, Ph.D., and his co-workers analyzed the phenol content of cocoa powder, dark chocolate, and milk chocolate and compared this to red wine. Dr. Waterhouse shows that one-and-a-half ounces of chocolate has the same amount of phenols as a five-ounce glass of red wine, and a cup of hot chocolate made with cocoa powder has about 75 percent of red wine's level.

These enologists also found that the phenols in chocolate behave the same way as those in red wine. Phenols protect the bad carriers of cholesterol, LDLs, from becoming damaging to artery walls by preventing the LDLs from oxidizing. And since oxidized LDLs are believed to be pivotal in the development of heart disease, anything that prevents this havoc helps reduce heart-disease risk.

There's more good news about chocolate. Despite chocolate's high fat content, with over 50 percent of chocolate's calories coming from fat and at least two-thirds coming from saturated fats, the type of fat in chocolate doesn't appear to raise blood cholesterol levels. Chocolate is rich in stearic acid, a type of saturated fat that leaves blood cholesterol levels alone.

All said and done, chocolate isn't as bad as you may have thought. But as with anything, moderation is the key. Most Americans eat on average just over 10 pounds of chocolate a year. (I am an above-average standout in this case.) Spread over a year's time, this amounts to less than half an ounce daily. So in the big picture, chocolate contributes little to our daily intake of calories and fat.

The bottom line for chocolate fans is to keep portion sizes small, and stick with dark chocolate which has a greater phenol content than milk chocolate. Or better yet, make hot chocolate with cocoa powder and nonfat milk. Here you get a dose of phenols (along with calcium) with only a speck of fat. By the way, white chocolate, which is not really chocolate at all, has no phenols.

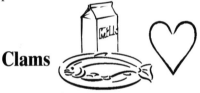

# Clams

Always keep canned clams on hand—these seafood wonders definitely ward off heart disease. A three-ounce serving of canned clams has only 126 calories and less than two grams of fat. But some of this fat is the omega-3 type that helps cut heart-disease risk. Also, clams are loaded with a staggering 4000 percent of your vitamin $B_{12}$ needs. This B vitamin works with other B vitamins such as folate and $B_6$ to keep homocysteine levels from becoming dangerous to your heart.

Besides all this, clams have about 60 milligrams of cholesterol, which may sound like bad news to you. But much of the "cholesterol" in clams are actually substances called *sterols* that actually block cholesterol absorption in the intestinal tract. In fact, eating clams on a regular basis may even lower blood cholesterol levels as a result of blocked absorption.

Researchers from the University of Washington in Seattle put clams to the test. Men with normal blood cholesterol levels were put on different diets of seafood to see if various shellfish have the power to lower blood cholesterol levels. Participants ate about a pound of fresh clams daily as their sole source of protein for a three-week test period. Compared to when they consumed their regular diet that included meat and eggs, blood cholesterol levels dropped. In fact, the level of the artery-clogging LDL cholesterol also fell.

The scientists then looked at how much of the dietary cholesterol absorption was blocked as a result of the sterols in clams. Evidence from this research reveals, that, when eaten regularly, clams block cholesterol absorption in the intestine enough to make an impact on blood cholesterol levels. This means clams make a great addition to your heart-healthy diet.

When purchasing fresh clams, freeze unless you plan to cook them the same day. Canned clams are decidedly easier to keep on hand and work well in chowders, seafood stews, casseroles, and dips. For a before-dinner, high-protein (but low-fat) dip with veggies, try mixing a package of nonfat cream cheese with fresh herbs (dill, parsley) and mix in a can of clams (drained). I often add a can or two of clams to ready-made canned clam chowder. This "beefs" up the protein content, providing half your daily requirement in a three-ounce serving of clams, and packs in heart-healthy ingredients. Try my recipe for quick Seafood Stew. Served with whole-grain bread, this hearty meal is welcome on a cold day.

### *Seafood Stew*

2 cans clams

2 oz. canned anchovies (optional)

6 to 8 oz. fresh catfish fillet, cut into bite-size chunks

1 can vegetable broth, low-sodium

2 med. Russet potatoes, cut into bite-size pieces

2 med. carrots, sliced

1 med. onion, chopped

2 cloves of garlic, crushed

1 med. tomato, chopped

1 bay leaf

fresh ground pepper

In a pot, sauté garlic and onions in 1 tablespoon of olive oil. Add carrot slices and potatoes and brown for another five minutes. Pour broth over vegetables, add bay leaf and ground pepper, then add enough water to cover potatoes. Bring to a boil and then turn down heat to let simmer until potatoes are soft but not mushy. Turn up heat and add catfish that has been cut into bite-size chunks; let simmer three minutes. Now add clams, anchovies, and chopped tomatoes. Cook another three to five minutes (do not overcook as this tends to toughen clams). Serves six.

| **Nutrition Facts** | |
|---|---|
| Seafood Stew | |
| Serving Size 1/6 recipe | |
| **Amount per Serving** | |
| Calories 223 | 36 Calories from fat |
| | % Daily Value |
| Total Fat 4g | 6% |
|    Saturated Fat <1g | 4% |
| Cholesterol 49mg | 16% |
| Sodium 960mg | 40% |
| Total Carbohydrate 23g | 8% |
|    Dietary Fiber 3g | 11% |
| Protein 23g | |
| Vitamin A 86%  •  Vitamin C 31% | |
| Calcium 9%  •  Iron 62% | |

# Coffee

Consider that almost 80 percent of Americans over the age of 20 drink coffee. You would think our coffee obsession started recently with the explosion in the number of coffee shops and espresso stands, but the seeds of this craving actually go back a thousand years or so. A dark slurry of ground coffee beans was made by the Arabs in Ethiopia around A.D. 1000. In fact, coffee is still enjoyed by many prepared that ancient way, Turkish style. Back then, as today, coffee drinkers enjoyed the stimulating effect of caffeine found naturally in coffee beans. In fact, we like coffee's wake-up call to the point that many of us are addicted to a daily dose of caffeine.

Is our habitual coffee-drinking "grounds" for concern when it comes to heart health? About 30 years ago researchers began snooping around for a possible coffee-and-heart-disease connection. Perhaps not surprisingly, researchers discovered that coffee drinkers appear to have a greater risk for heart attacks than nondrinkers.

Yet the scientific evidence wasn't solid; some studies found no ill effects of Java. Some of the conflicting results were due to the fact that many heavy coffee drinkers are also smokers, which unto its own, causes heart disease. But this didn't explain why even among nonsmokers, heart-disease risk appeared linked to coffee-drinking under certain conditions.

### Brewing Trouble

Scientists noticed that European research studies tended to find a link between coffee drinking and heart attacks while studies here in the U.S. failed to find this connection. Why the difference? Coffee brewing methods typically used in Europe, such as boiled or espresso coffee, may be to blame.

According to new research, coffee beans contain substances that raise blood cholesterol levels. These chemicals, called *cafestol* and *kahweol,* are found in coffee oils which can be leached out into the coffee depending on how it is brewed. Cafestol and kahweol end up in the brew when the coffee grounds come in contact with boiling hot water. Boiled coffee (grounds combined with boiling water and allowed to steep), espresso, plunger pot coffee (often called *cafetiére* coffee), and Turkish coffee are all prepared in this way. And it makes no difference if the coffee beans are decaf or regular, both contain coffee oils with cafestol and kahweol.

Drip coffee, however, is free of these coffee nasties. When coffee runs through a filter, cafestol and kahweol get trapped in the filter paper. So drip coffee, most commonly served in restaurants and homes here, has virtually no cafestol or kahweol. This helps explain why researchers in the U.S. didn't find a consistent connection between coffee drinking and heart attack risk. Coffee made from instant is also low in these harmful substances. Researchers were surprised to find out that percolated coffee is also low in cafestol and kahweol despite the fact it comes in direct contact with the coffee grounds without a filter.

Cafestol and kahweol are not lightweights when it comes to tampering with blood cholesterol levels. Studies show that a regular intake of these coffee bad guys can raise cholesterol levels significantly. To add to the bad news, cafestol and kahweol boost LDL levels, the cholesterol carrier that blocks arteries. In fact, several studies show that regular intake of cafestol and kahweol, the amount found in about five cups of Turkish brewed coffee, can raise LDL levels by a dangerous 25 percent. Of course, I have never met anyone who desires five cups of this seriously thick brew.

### Go Easy on the Caffeine

In addition to boosting blood cholesterol levels, coffee drinking may also spell trouble for people at risk for high blood pressure. In one study, researchers showed that young men at risk for high blood pressure (that is, at least one parent was hypertensive) may be more sensitive to caffeine's stimulatory effect by raising blood pressure. The study participants were tested under a mentally stressful situation following a dose of caffeine equal to two to three cups of coffee. Researchers found elevated levels of the stress hormone *cortisol,* which causes blood pressure to rise. Other studies show that caffeine causes blood pressure numbers to rise in people already diagnosed with hypertension.

So if high blood pressure plagues you, or if you may be at risk, keep caffeine consumption to a minimum. Ask your physician about interaction of caffeine and other medications you may be taking in the event excessive caffeine intake may change the effectiveness of your drugs. Also, monitor your level of mental stress—change in jobs, family troubles, etc. This type of stress may aggravate caffeine's effect on your blood pressure.

### Coffee Talk

Where does all this talk about blood cholesterol and high blood pressure leave us coffee drinkers? Researchers are still not in agreement whether coffee is truly detrimental to your heart, especially when compared to other culprits such as eating too much fat. But enough evidence exists to warn java junkies that moderating their coffee consumption may well be in their heart's best interest.

How much coffee is considered "not too much"? Most coffee/heart disease researchers agree that in excess of five cups of drip, instant, or percolated coffee per day warrants some cautions, particularly if blood cholesterol levels are in the risky range and/or blood pressure is on the rise. Also, if multiple cappuccinos, caffé lattes, and mochas (all made with espresso) make their way into your daily fare, cutting back to one a day would be advised.

Here are some ways to cut back on your coffee and caffeine consumption without giving up the ship.

- If you are a true "caffeine head" drinking several cups of coffee daily, avoid going cold turkey. Instead, ease back by cutting one cup every few weeks. This helps avoid possible caffeine withdrawal troubles such as headache and feelings of fatigue.

- Try substituting some decaffeinated grounds for regular when making coffee. Start off slowly by replacing less than one-fourth the grounds with decaf. Then increase the proportion of decaf every few weeks.

## Beware of Beverages

Watch for hidden calories and caffeine in your favorite drinks.

| Beverages | Calories | Fat (gm) | Caffeine (mg) |
|---|---|---|---|
| *Coffee* | | | |
| Brewed, 6 oz. | 4 | 0 | 103 |
| Instant, decaf, 6 oz. | 4 | 0 | 2 |
| | | | |
| *Espresso, 4 oz.* | 0 | 0 | 102 |
| Low-fat Mocha,* 12 oz. | 300 | 17 | 102 |
| Nonfat Mocha,* 12 oz. | 260 | 11 | 102 |
| Low-fat Latte,* 12 oz. | 170 | 6 | 102 |
| Nonfat Latte,* 12 oz. | 120 | <1 | 102 |
| | | | |
| *Tea* | | | |
| Black, 6 oz. | 2 | 0 | 53 |
| Herb, 6 oz. | 1 | 0 | 32 |
| Iced tea, instant, 8 oz. | 1 | 0 | 30 |
| | | | |
| *Soda, 12 fl. oz.* | | | |
| Mountain Dew | 179 | 0 | 55 |
| Coca-Cola | 154 | 0 | 47 |
| Pepsi | 190 | 0 | 37 |
| Diet Pepsi | 0 | 0 | 37 |
| Slice | 152 | 0 | 11 |
| | | | |
| *Bottled Water, 12 oz.* | | | |
| Java Water | 0 | 0 | 71 |

*Source:* Bowes & Church's *Food Values of Portions Commonly Used,* 17th ed., Lippincott, 1998.

* Starbucks coffee (fat from chocolate mix)

### What's Brewing

Coffee brews and levels of cafestol and kahweol.

| *Low* | *Medium* | *High* |
|---|---|---|
| Drip coffee | Espresso | Plunger pot coffee |
| Percolated coffee | Instant | Turkish/Greek coffee |

- Avoid drinking sodas as a "coffee" alternative. Many sodas such as colas have added caffeine. In addition, you may get some unwanted sugar calories if you down non-diet varieties. Check the "Beware of Beverages" chart for caffeine and calorie levels in many beverages.

- Fill up your coffee mug with fresh water and a twist of lemon; you may find this satisfying and even more refreshing than a cup of joe.

- If you use coffee to fight fatigue, especially at work, instead try getting up from your chair and taking a walk around the office, getting some fresh air, or doing some simple stretches at your work place. This bit of activity may snap you out of your daze without the help of caffeine.

# Corn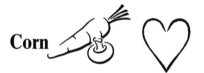

What would summer be like without farm-fresh corn-on-the-cob? When you bite into an ear of sweet corn, you not only get a taste of summer but also some unexpected goodness for your heart. What may be an annoyance—the kernel skins that get stuck in your teeth—is actually a heart saver. These skins contain corn bran, a fiber that has been shown to lower blood cholesterol levels.

Researchers from Illinois State University put corn bran to the test in a group of men with risky levels of blood cholesterol.

After a few weeks on a low-fat diet, the men were given 20 grams daily of either corn bran mixed with their food or the same amount of wheat bran (the fiber from wheat). Following six weeks of bran boosted diets, the men's cholesterol levels were tested again. Cholesterol levels dropped only in those men eating the corn bran. These results give good reason to include corn or other corn products such as whole cornmeal or corn grits (made from whole kernels of corn) in your diet.

One medium sized ear of corn has about three grams of fiber and only 80 calories. A half cup of cooked corn grits or quarter cup of cornmeal (raw) used in muffins or bread has about the same amount of fiber. And that's not all. Fresh corn is a good source of folate. One ear has almost 20 percent of your daily needs. This B vitamin helps clear homocysteine, a blood metabolite that causes damage to artery walls.

Buy fresh corn in season for best flavor and nutrition. Look for ears still in their husk. Husks can be left on for cooking corn on the grill—simply pull back the husks, remove the silk, and spray or rinse the corn with water. Then unfold the husks to cover the corn and grill until tender, about 10 minutes. Besides eating straight off the cob, corn makes a great addition to cold salads or in hot dishes including casseroles or soups. My Corn-Pepper Salad (recipe follows) makes a great side dish for fish. Frozen corn makes a convenient substitution for fresh and still has all the great nutrition.

Cornmeal and grits can be used in baked goods or as a cooked cereal. Select whole corn meal or grits as the refined versions have little cholesterol-lowering fiber. You can also purchase corn bran, much richer in fiber than whole corn meal or grits. Check your supermarket or local health food store for corn bran. Use corn bran as a cooked cereal or add to your favorite cornbread recipe for a fiber boost. Some ready-to-eat breakfast cereals also have added corn bran. Check the ingredient label and Nutrition Facts panel for fiber content.

### *Corn-Pepper Salad*

8 ears of corn (par boiled)

2 red and 2 green bell peppers, seeds removed and diced into small pieces

juice from 4 limes

1 hot pepper (sereno or jalapeño)

1/3 cup chopped fresh coriander

Cut the corn off the cob and place into a bowl. Add diced peppers and lime juice, toss until mixed. Finely dice hot pepper (careful not to touch eyes during this as it may irritate) and add to corn mixture along with chopped coriander. Serves eight.

| **Nutrition Facts** |
| --- |
| Corn-Pepper Salad |
| Serving Size 1/8 recipe |

| Amount per Serving | |
| --- | --- |
| Calories 88 | 9 Calories from fat |

| | % Daily Value |
| --- | --- |
| Total Fat 1g | 1% |
|    Saturated Fat 0g | 0% |
| Cholesterol 0mg | 0% |
| Sodium 20mg | 1% |
| Total Carbohydrate 21g | 7% |
|    Dietary Fiber 4g | 16% |
| Protein 3g | |

| | | |
| --- | --- | --- |
| Vitamin A 6% | • | Vitamin C 85% |
| Calcium 1% | • | Iron 4% |
| | • | Vitamin $B_6$ 15% |

# Crackers

We snack on them right out of the box, crumble a few over hot soup, and even make a meal out of several topped with cheese. Crackers are fun to munch. If you choose the right ones, you can get some energizing carbohydrates, B vitamins, and fiber for heart health while you're snacking away. But finding healthful crackers can be tricky. Many come loaded with unwanted fat and sodium, while others lead you to believe that they are nutritious with names like "Multi-Grain," "7-Grain Stone Ground," "Reduced-Fat," and "Fat-Free."

Choosing the right cracker as part of your Simple Six Eating Plan takes a little bit of "cracker" savvy. Here's a buyer's guide to get you started along with a chart on top crackers and toppings for your cracker selection.

### Cracker Buyer's Guide

When navigating the cracker aisle at your grocery store, do some label reading before you buy.

- *Check the serving size.* A serving of crackers is usually one ounce, but this could mean one cracker to 30 crackers depending on the brand. Before you start munching right out of the box, remove one serving then close the box. This way you can keep a lid on how much you eat.

- *Check the fat content.* Select crackers that have no more than three grams of fat per serving. Keep in mind that "reduced-fat" crackers may still have more fat than you bargained for.

- *Watch out for sodium.* Most crackers are salty—some have more than 300 to 400 milligrams in a serving. Select those with a sodium count less than 200 milligrams per serving.

- *Find the fiber.* Crackers have anywhere from zero to over 6 grams of fiber per serving. Select a cracker that has at least 2 or more grams. Don't let names like "7-Grain" lead you into believing this cracker also is packed with fiber. Many crackers list refined flour as their first ingredient making them marginal on fiber. Look for crackers made with 100 percent whole-grain flour as one of the first ingredients.

- *Avoid hydrogenated fats.* Crackers made with added fat often have hydrogenated fats as part of their ingredient list. This means un-wanted artery-clogging saturated and *trans* fats. When buying a cracker with added fat, look for unprocessed oils on the ingredient list.

# Cracker Comparison

Here's how some cracker favorites stack up.

| Cracker | Serving Size | Calories | Fat (gm) | Fiber (gm) | Sodium (mg) |
|---|---|---|---|---|---|
| Devonsheer Plain Melba Rounds | 10 crackers | 100 | 0 | 2 | 190 |
| Nabisco Fat-Free Premium Saltines | 10 crackers | 120 | 0 | 0 | 360 |
| Snackwell's Fat-Free Wheat | 10 crackers | 120 | 0 | 2 | 340 |
| Snackwell's Fat-Free Cracked Pepper | 14 crackers | 120 | 0 | 1 | 300 |
| Nabisco Reduced-Fat Triscuit | 8 crackers | 130 | 3 | 4 | 180 |
| Nabisco Harvest Crisps | 13 crackers | 130 | 3.5 | 1 | 270 |
| Nabisco Reduced-Fat Wheat Thins | 18 crackers | 120 | 4 | 2 | 220 |
| Nabisco Reduced-Fat Ritz | 10 crackers | 140 | 4 | 0 | 280 |
| Sunshine Reduced-Fat Cheez-it | 29 crackers | 140 | 4.5 | <1 | 280 |
| Pepperidge Farm Goldfish | 55 pieces | 140 | 6 | <1 | 240 |
| Sunshine Cheez-it | 13 crackers | 150 | 8 | <1 | 230 |
| Nabisco Ritz | 10 crackers | 160 | 8 | 0 | 270 |

*Source:* Manufacturers' Food Labels

## Tops on the List

Try these spreads and toppings as healthful additions to your crackers.

| Serving (2 tbsp.) | Fat (grams) | Calories |
|---|---|---|
| Apple Butter | 0 | 90 |
| Fruit Spread | 0 | 90 |
| Fat-Free Cheese (1 oz.) | 0 | 45 |
| Fat-Free Cream Cheese | 0 | 30 |
| Low-Fat Hummus | 2 | 45 |
| Salsa | 0 | 10 |
| Reduced-Fat Goat Cheese | 3 | 65 |

*Source:* Manufacturers' Food Labels

# Cranberries

This fruit, traditionally made into sauce for the holidays, may be one of the best disease-fighting foods on your overloaded turkey-day plate. Cranberries' rich color comes from a type of flavonoid called *rhamnoside*. Like other flavonoids found in wine and tea, rhamnoside acts as an antioxidant. Antioxidants like this help fend off heart disease by protecting LDLs (cholesterol bad guys) from becoming damaged and infiltrating artery walls.

Many studies show that people who have a high intake of flavonoids, also found in onions, apples, and other vegetables and fruits, have a lower risk for heart disease and stroke. In one study, over 500 men were tracked for 15 years. Scientists evaluated the men's intake of flavonoids and found that those men with a low intake were about 70 percent more likely to suffer from stroke compared to those with the highest flavonoid intake.

So load up your plate with cranberry sauce this Thanksgiving. You can cut back on some of the added sugar in commercial sauce by making your own. Put fresh cranberries in a pot and add enough water to keep them from sticking to the bottom of the pan as you cook them. Then add orange juice concentrate for sweetener at the end. You can also use dried cranberries as a topping to your morning cereal, add to trail mix (see my recipe on page 54), or just eat plain—their tangy zing can be habit forming.

# Dates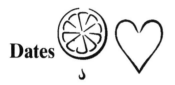

Make a date with a date soon. This delectably sweet fruit helps fight hypertension and keeps your heart healthy. Actually a berry with a rigid seed on the inside, dates pack a duo of high blood pressure fighting nutrients—fiber and potassium. A serving of about 10 medium sized dates supplies a generous 25 percent of your fiber needs along with about 600 milligrams or 15 percent of your daily potassium needs. According to studies from around the world, the fiber and potassium in fruit may work in concert to fend off hypertension.

In one study from the Department of Epidemiology, Harvard School of Public Health in Boston, scientists studied the relationship of fruit consumption and its possible blood pressure lowering benefits. Over 800 men were examined for their intake of fruit servings daily as well as other dietary factors and blood pressure readings. The researchers found that men eating a fruit-rich diet had lower blood pressure readings than men who consumed little fruit. In fact, the scientists determined that for each additional serving of fruit daily, blood pressure dropped by a small but significant amount.

While harvested from date palm trees during the fall months, dates are available in packaged form year round. You can purchase dates with or without the seed, or pit, as well as chopped. Avoid dates that look overly dry or cracked. Due to their low moisture content, dates keep for months if refrigerated in a well-sealed container.

There are a million ways to make a date with dates. Add them to just about anything for a dose of sweetness to go with your fiber and potassium. Top off your cereal with chopped dates, fill whole dates with an almond or walnut half for a sweet nutty crunch, mix chopped dates into a fruit salad, or add to cookie dough, muffin batter, or bread recipes. Dates and nuts pureed together in a food processor make a great topping for whole-grain pancakes. Also try dates with vegetables, rice, beans, or meats. Jazz up a pot of brown rice by stirring in a handful of chopped dates. After the rice is fully cooked, add dates and allow a few minutes for steaming, then serve. Try my Date-Cashew Rice dish for a taste adventure that's good for your heart.

### *Date-Cashew Rice*

10 large dates, chopped

1 large onion, chopped

1 tsp. fresh ginger, finely chopped

2 cups rice (brown or white)

3 cups water

1 tbsp. canola oil

1/2 cup chopped unsalted cashews

In a saucepan, heat oil and sauté over medium heat the onion, ginger, and dates until the onion is soft. Add rice and water, stir, and then cover saucepan. Turn down heat to medium-low and cook for 20 minutes or until rice is done. Garnish with chopped cashews. Makes eight servings.

**Nutrition Facts**

Date-Cashew Rice

Serving Size 1/8 recipe

| Amount per Serving | |
| --- | --- |
| Calories 266 | 54 Calories from fat |

| | % Daily Value |
| --- | --- |
| Total Fat 6g | 9% |
| Saturated Fat 1g | 5% |
| Cholesterol 0mg | 0% |
| Sodium 5mg | 0% |
| Total Carbohydrate 48g | 16% |
| Dietary Fiber 2g | 8% |
| Protein 5g | |

| | | |
| --- | --- | --- |
| Vitamin A 0% | • | Vitamin C 1% |
| Calcium 2% | • | Iron 17% |
| | • | Vitamin E 13% |

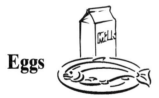

# Eggs

Sure, an egg is loaded with cholesterol. But don't let that stop you from enjoying this nutrient powerhouse. Mounting research shows eating three or four eggs weekly or even as many as one or two daily is okay for your heart. In fact, contrary to popular belief, scientific studies failed to link egg consumption with heart disease or hypertension in the first place. The egg scare got its start when researchers first connected high blood cholesterol levels to heart-disease risk. Unfortunately, eggs became guilty by association.

We need to remember that for most of us, *dietary* cholesterol from eggs and other foods does not have an impact on our *blood* cholesterol levels. About three-fourths of the population is able to gear down their production of cholesterol to compensate for what is coming in the body from foods.

Bumping eggs out of your diet in hopes of lowering heart-disease risk may actually be a bad idea. Eggs are packed with good nutrition. One large egg has only 75 calories and five grams of fat with about half of this from heart-healthy monounsaturated fats. Eggs also contain nature's best protein source along with other nutrients including folate, riboflavin, vitamins A and $B_{12}$; and they are one of the few dietary sources of vitamin D. Since eggs are so nutrient dense, they become a must for people eating very little, such as the elderly and those cutting back on calories for weight loss.

Some specialty brands of eggs are now available that come pumped up with even more good nutrition especially for your heart. For example, a Texas-based egg producer, Pilgrim Pride, now sells eggs that deliver about 60 percent of vitamin E needs, good for protecting LDLs from damaging artery walls. These eggs also provide 100 milligrams of omega-3 fats, typically not found in eggs, which also help protect against heart disease. As an added bonus, research shows that these omega-3-boosted eggs will actually lower blood fat levels. Feeding the hens a special diet that includes flax seed which is rich in omega-3 fats gives these specialty eggs their nutritional boost. These super eggs taste, cook, and look like ordinary ones.

### Good Eggs

Let me convince you that if you were eating eggs on a regular basis you are not the "bad egg" you once thought. In one study, men were fed either three, seven, or 14 eggs per week for five months. Following this egg treatment, blood cholesterol levels were measured along with other risk factors for heart disease. Despite heavy egg consumption amounting to an extra 220 to 440 milligrams of cholesterol daily, none of the men showed an increase in blood cholesterol levels.

Along the same lines, here's a true story I want to share with you. An 88-year-old man was reported to eat an average of 15 to

25 eggs daily (and that's no yolk!). He practiced his egg-eating routine for 15 years and suffered no ill effects. His blood cholesterol levels were healthy. While I'm not suggesting you gobble down 15 eggs a day, you certainly can include eggs in your weekly or even daily menu.

### Egg Alternatives

For those individuals who have dangerously high blood cholesterol levels and cutting back on dietary cholesterol is a must, consider egg substitutes. Provided you like your eggs scrambled, these products are a fabulous trade-off for the real thing (see "Egg Stats" chart for comparison). Egg substitutes are fat and cholesterol free, a great source of protein (made mostly from egg whites) along with folate, riboflavin, and vitamins A and $B_{12.}$ Use egg substitutes the same way you would regular eggs in omelets, casseroles, baked goods, French toast, desserts, and anything else you can think of.

An advantage of egg substitutes over the real thing is that they are pasteurized, meaning heat treated, so there is no risk of food poisoning from salmonella bacteria found in raw eggs. For any recipe that calls for uncooked eggs, you can safely use egg substitutes. Also, egg substitutes can be frozen (find some brands in the frozen foods section of your supermarket).

### Egg Stats

| Types of Eggs | Calories | Fat (gm) | Saturated Fat (gm) | Cholesterol (mg) |
|---|---|---|---|---|
| Whole egg | 75 | 5 | 1.5 | 213 |
| Egg yolk | 59 | 5 | 1.5 | 213 |
| Egg white | 17 | 0 | 0 | 0 |
| Egg beaters | 30 | 0 | 0 | 0 |

*Source:* Manufacturers' Food Label

## Fabulous Vanilla French Toast

4 hearty slices of whole-grain sourdough bread

3/4 cup egg substitute or 2 whole eggs + 2 egg whites

3 tbsp. milk

1/2 tsp. vanilla

1/2 tsp. cinnamon

dash allspice

Combine all the ingredients (except the bread) in a bowl. Whisk the mixture until light and fluffy (about 2 minutes). Dip one slice of bread at a time on both sides making sure to cover all edges. Place in a heated nonstick skillet and brown on both sides. If using whole eggs, cook thoroughly. Top with fresh sliced strawberries and a dollop of vanilla nonfat yogurt. Makes four servings.

| **Nutrition Facts** | |
| :--- | ---: |
| Fabulous Vanilla French Toast* | |
| Serving Size 1 slice | |
| **Amount per Serving** | |
| Calories 211  34 Calories from fat | |
| | % Daily Value |
| Total Fat 4g | 6% |
|    Saturated Fat 1g | 4% |
| Cholesterol 0mg | 0% |
| Sodium 324mg | 13% |
| Total Carbohydrate 32g | 11% |
|    Dietary Fiber 5g | 20% |
| Protein 12g | |
| Vitamin A 13%  •  Vitamin C 71% | |
| Calcium 16%  •  Iron 16% | |

* (with strawberries and yogurt topping)

# Eggplant

With its satin smooth purple finish, I often display eggplant on my kitchen counter, besides eating it for heart health. It is actually that beautiful purple color that gives eggplant its heart saving qualities. The phytochemical *nasunin,* which is a type of purple pigment found in other vegetables and fruits like red cabbage and grapes, has been shown to help lower blood cholesterol levels. Besides nasunin, eggplant is also a great source of potassium to help fight high blood pressure. And as an extra bonus, a half-cup cooked serving also supplies about seven percent of folate and fiber needs all in just 13 calories.

Researchers from Yamagata University in Japan studied the effect of dosing laboratory animals with eggplant's nasunin while the animals ate a diet loaded with cholesterol. The scientists wanted to know if nasunin was effective in lowering the animals' blood cholesterol levels. They were also checking on whether nasunin could block the absorption of cholesterol into the body.

After a few weeks on the high-cholesterol diet with nasunin, the animals' blood cholesterol levels dropped compared to a group that did not get the nasunin. There's more good news: HDL levels went up in the group getting the nasunin. More HDLs can mean lower risk for heart disease since these cholesterol carriers help rid the body of unwanted cholesterol. Also, the researchers found that the nasunin was blocking absorption of cholesterol from the diet because more cholesterol was appearing in the animals' waste.

So help yourself to some eggplant. But one word of caution: Eggplant's unusual cell structure makes it a great "sponge," especially for oil. This means if you cook eggplant in a pan with some oil, the eggplant soaks the oil up just like a sponge. The best way to cook eggplant is in bite-size pieces or sliced in an oven casserole. You can also microwave eggplant until tender and top it with a small amount of shaved Parmesan cheese. Eggplant is also a great addition to Indian curries and is most popular in a vegetable medley called *ratatouille*.

## Japanese Eggplant with Ginger

5 Japanese eggplant (about 5 to 7 inches long), sliced in 1/4-inch rounds

5 cloves of garlic, sliced

1 tbsp. dry black salted beans (available at Asian food market or section in grocery store)

1 tbsp. diced fresh ginger

2 tsp. canola oil

1/2 cup water

1/2 bunch of scallions, chopped

In a skillet or wok with cover, heat oil over medium heat. Add garlic, ginger, and salted black beans and sauté lightly. Add sliced eggplant and water and cook until eggplant is soft (cover to steam eggplant). Just before serving, toss with scallions as a garnish. Serves eight.

| **Nutrition Facts** | |
| :--- | ---: |
| Japanese Eggplant with Ginger | |
| Serving Size 1/8 recipe | |
| **Amount per Serving** | |
| Calories 45        16 Calories from fat | |
| | % Daily Value |
| Total Fat 2g | 3% |
| Saturated Fat 0g | 0% |
| Cholesterol 0mg | 0% |
| Sodium 272mg | 11% |
| Total Carbohydrate 7g | 2% |
| Dietary Fiber 3g | 13% |
| Protein 1g | |
| Vitamin A 1%   •   Vitamin C 5% | |
| Calcium 4%   •   Iron 4% | |

# Fat-Free Cookies

While even I hate to admit it, cookies certainly don't offer much in the way of heart-healthy ingredients. Consider the basics that go into a batch of cookies: butter, sugar, eggs, and flour. Perhaps some raisins, nuts, or oatmeal may be tossed in, but usually not enough to have any redeeming qualities. Each cookie can easily average 5 to 10 grams of fat, and usually this fat is mostly artery-clogging saturated fat.

For cookie-monster types (like myself), fat-free cookies and reduced-fat versions offer a tasty alternative. But eater beware: Fat-free cookies still have calories so eating a handful can easily add to your waist if you're not careful. And reduced-fat cookies may not be much of a fat savings at all since "reduced-fat" simply means 25 percent less fat than the regular version. Some brands of reduced-fat chocolate chip cookies, for example, still have over five grams of fat per serving.

If you can't resist dipping your hand into the cookie jar, that's okay. You can easily fit certain cookies into the Simple Six Eating Plan without risking your heart health. Use these tips when selecting cookies. Also, in the "Look What's in the Cookie Jar" chart, I list some great selections along with a few best left on the shelf.

### Tips for a Cookie Monster

- Look at the Nutrition Facts food label first; select cookies that have less than four grams of fat per serving. And note that serving sizes vary depending on the size of the cookies.
- Check the ingredient list for the type of fat used in baking. Avoid hydrogenated fats as these contain artery-damaging *trans* fats. Most cookies contain saturated fat as well, more reason to select fat-free cookies.

## Look What's in the Cookie Jar

Here's a selection of low-fat and fat-free cookies, along with a few that are best left in the cookie jar.

| Cookies | Serving Size | Calories | Fat (gm) | Sugar (gm) | Fiber (gm) | Sodium (mg) |
|---|---|---|---|---|---|---|
| Healthy Valley Fat-Free Chocolate Chip | 3 cookies | 100 | 0 | 10 | 3 | 40 |
| Snackwell's Devil's Food Cookie Cakes | 1 cookie | 50 | 0 | 9 | 0 | 30 |
| Snackwell's Reduced-Fat Oatmeal Raisin | 2 cookies | 110 | 2.5 | 10 | 1 | 135 |
| Nabisco Fig Newtons | 2 cookies | 110 | 2.5 | 14 | 1 | 125 |
| Pepperidge Farm Milano | 2 cookies | 130 | 7 | 8 | <1 | 65 |
| Mother's Cookie Parade | 4 cookies | 140 | 7 | 9 | 2 | 95 |
| Nabisco Oreo | 3 cookies | 160 | 7 | 13 | 1 | 220 |
| Nabisco Reduced-Fat Oreo | 3 cookies | 130 | 3.5 | 14 | 1 | 190 |
| Nabisco Nilla Wafers | 8 wafers | 140 | 5 | 12 | 0 | 100 |
| Nabisco Reduced Fat Nilla Wafers | 8 wafers | 120 | 2 | 12 | 0 | 105 |
| Nabisco Reduced Fat Chips Ahoy! | 3 cookies | 140 | 5 | 10 | <1 | 150 |
| Nabisco Honey Maid Graham Crackers | 8 crackers | 120 | 3 | 7 | 1 | 180 |
| Nabisco Low-Fat Honey Maid Graham Crackers | 8 crackers | 110 | 1.5 | 8 | <1 | 200 |

*Source:* Manufacturers' Food Labels

- Surprisingly many cookies come with a big dose of unwanted sodium. Select those with less than about 120 milligrams per serving.

- Sugar is bound to be on the ingredient list. Keep in mind that four grams of sugar is equal to one teaspoon. Since sugar has no nutritional value and may raise blood fat levels in some people, you're better off selecting a cookie with less than seven grams, or one and a half teaspoons of sugar.

- Don't be swayed by cookies made with "natural" sweeteners like white grape juice concentrate. Whether the sugar used is plain old white table sugar, honey, or anything else, they are all sugar with no extra nutritional boost.

- Some cookies actually have some nutritional benefits. Those cookies made with real fruit like Fig Newtons or with 100 percent whole-wheat flour most likely will contain a few grams of fiber. Check the label and ingredient list and know that product names such as "natural" and "whole wheat" don't guarantee you better nutrition.

# Figs

Most of us know a fig for its well-known leaf cover-up used by Adam and Eve. Just like the fig leaf, the use of the fig's fruit dates back to prehistoric times, but it is "designed" more like a high-tech food of today. Figs have a nutritional profile unlike most fruits, almost as if they were created for heart health. Figs come packed with a wealth of minerals and fiber helpful in fighting hypertension and high blood cholesterol. In fact, they are a must for people serious about keeping hypertension at bay.

The power trio, as I call them—potassium, calcium, and magnesium—come together in figs as a virtual arsenal against hypertension. Researchers have long noted that many people with high blood pressure, notoriously men, eat diets marginal in these minerals. And a recent study involving both men and women showed that eating foods rich in these three minerals helps lower blood pressure as effectively as drugs.

Most fruits provide little in the way of calcium or magnesium but supply a modest amount of potassium. But figs pack as much potassium as a banana and contain about 10 percent of calcium and magnesium needs in just one serving of four dried figs. You'd have to eat a hefty serving of collard greens for that kind of nutrition.

Figs are also an outstanding source of fiber—a whopping nine grams in one serving. Most of this fiber is the water-soluble type which helps lower blood cholesterol levels by blocking the absorption of cholesterol in the intestines. Other fruits also have fiber, but figs contain at least two to three times as much fiber per serving as most fruits. In fact, calorie for calorie, figs have more fiber than apples or raisins. In fact, a serving of figs has more fiber than a bowl of raisin bran cereal!

Select fresh figs that are free of any major skin blemishes. Or for the ultimate in convenience, dried figs come in resealable plastic bags for quick, delicious snacking and lasting freshness. Use fresh figs within about four to six days and dried within about two to three months, and store both in the refrigerator. Dried or fresh figs make a great anytime snack. I like to use figs as a sweet treat before a workout or as a pick-me-up at work. You can use chopped figs in muffin recipes, or as a topping for nonfat vanilla yogurt.

# Flax Seed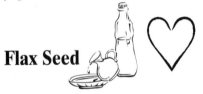

Not just for eating, the versatility of flax and its seed is absolutely amazing. An infusion made with flax seed has been used for centuries as a styling gel in women's hair. Flax fibers are woven into a linen-like cloth, and flax seed oil (a.k.a. linseed oil) is used in furniture varnishes and cleaners. So how could this almost industrial-sounding plant seed have anything to offer your heart? Flax seed comes packed with the same heart-healthy oils as fish: omega-3 fats. And to boot, flax seed is a great source of fiber as well as calcium to help lower high blood pressure.

Flax seeds, a dark brown version of sesame seeds, contain about nine grams of fat in a one-ounce serving. But over half of the fat is alpha-linolenic acid which is the plant form of omega-3 fats, the same sought-after fat found in salmon, sardines, and other fish as well as those fish oil capsules many of us take. Flax seeds' high content of omega-3s is big news since canola and walnut oil are a distant second place with less than 10 percent of their fat as alpha-linolenic acid. For nonfish eaters or vegetarians, flax seed is your best bet in getting these heart-healthy fats.

Omega-3 fats keep blood cells called *platelets* from becoming sticky, which helps prevent blood clots from forming in narrowed arteries. Also, omega-3s help lower blood fat levels. In one study, subjects with risky blood cholesterol levels ate bread made with ground flax seed for three months. Participants ate three slices of bread daily containing 15 grams of ground flax seed. Following "bread" therapy, the participants' cholesterol levels dropped dramatically, especially levels of the "bad" cholesterol LDL. Also, the patients' platelets were less sticky following flax seed consumption.

The oil in flax seed may also provide some benefit for rigid arteries that develop as a result of poor health conditions such as diabetes and obesity. In one study, overweight subjects used a margarine made with flax seed oil in place of regular margarine. Following four weeks of treatment, the elasticity of the participants' blood vessels improved.

Apparently flax seeds work, but you might think they taste more like bird seed (not that I've eaten bird seed lately). You will be pleasantly surprised. Fix yourself a flax seed muffin—it tastes great. According to an official taste test comparing flax seed muffins with standard muffins, tasters preferred the muffins made with flax seeds. You'll love my tried-and-true recipe for ground flax seed muffins.

But note that when making these muffins, you must either purchase ground flax seeds (called flax seed meal) or grind them yourself in a coffee grinder. The outer covering of unground flax seeds is pretty tough and will go right through your system undigested. So if you're after a laxative, use whole flax seeds; otherwise, to get the heart-healthy oils, use ground flax seed. Also, take

## What's All the Flax About?

Here are a few ready-to-eat breakfast cereals made with flax seeds.

| | | | |
|---|---|---|---|
| Healthy Valley Golden Flax Cereal *serving size 1/2 cup* | 190 calories | 6 grams of fiber | 1000 mg of Omega-3 |
| Lifestream Flax Plus *serving size 3/4 cup* | 120 calories | 5 grams of fiber | 400 mg of Omega-3 |
| Nature's Path Mesa Sunrise *serving size 3/4 cup* | 130 calories | 2 grams of fiber | 300 mg of Omega-3 |

a look at the ready-to-eat breakfast cereals that are made with flax seed meal.

Make sure to store flax seed in the refrigerator as the fats easily go bad. You can also purchase flax seed oil at health food stores. Use this in salad dressings, tossed with cooked pasta, or drizzled on pizza. It's important to note that flax seed oil cannot be used in cooking because at high temperatures the beneficial oils break down.

### *Flax Seed Buttermilk Muffins*

1 cup flour

1/2 cup whole-wheat flour

1/2 cup flax seed meal (use coffee grinder to process flax seed)

1/2 cup quick oats

2 tsp. baking powder

1/2 tsp. baking soda

1/2 cup egg substitute (or two eggs)

1 cup buttermilk

4 tbsp. honey

2/3 cup raisins

Mix all dry ingredients together in a bowl. Combine liquid ingredients in a separate bowl (keep raisins in reserve). Stir liquid ingredients into dry ingredients all at once, add raisins, and stir until thoroughly moistened but the batter still appears lumpy. Fill muffin tins lined with paper or foil cups about two-thirds full. Bake at 400 degrees for 20 to 25 minutes. Serve topped with jam.

## Nutrition Facts

Flax Seed Buttermilk Muffins

Serving Size 1 muffin

| Amount per Serving | |
| --- | --- |
| Calories 165 | 27 Calories from fat |
| | % Daily Value |
| Total Fat 3g | 5% |
| Saturated Fat <.5g | 1% |
| Cholesterol 0mg | 0% |
| Sodium 76mg | 3% |
| Total Carbohydrate 30g | 10% |
| Dietary Fiber 3g | 12% |
| Protein 6g | |

| | | |
| --- | --- | --- |
| Vitamin A 3% | • | Vitamin C 1% |
| Calcium 9% | • | Iron 13% |

# Frozen Dinners

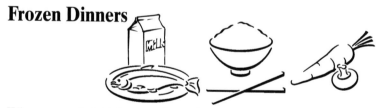

When you get right down to it, each year you scramble for a dinner 365 times. Let's say you eat out at least once a week; that still leaves about 300 dinners you need to create. Thank goodness for frozen dinners. Ready anytime you are, frozen dinners are convenient and 'wave up in a matter of minutes. As for taste, many of

## Frozen and Delicious

Here's a sampling of some low-fat entrées and meals available in your frozen foods aisle.

| Meal | Calories | Fat (gm) | Fiber (gm) | Cholesterol (mg) | Sodium (mg) |
|---|---|---|---|---|---|
| *Chicken* | | | | | |
| Healthy Choice Country Glazed Chicken | 220 | 3 | 3 | 40 | 480 |
| Healthy Choice Chicken and Vegetable Marsala | 230 | 1.5 | 3 | 30 | 440 |
| Healthy Choice Chicken Parmigiana | 330 | 8 | 4 | 40 | 490 |
| Lean Cuisine Chicken Picata | 270 | 6 | 2 | 25 | 530 |
| Lean Cuisine Grilled Chicken Salsa | 270 | 7 | 4 | 45 | 570 |
| Lean Cuisine Herb Roasted Chicken | 210 | 5 | 3 | 40 | 540 |
| Michelina's Chicken Primavera with Spirals | 250 | 7 | 2 | 35 | 860 |
| Smart Ones Honey Mustard Chicken | 200 | 2 | 3 | 30 | 370 |
| *Beef* | | | | | |
| Healthy Choice Salisbury Steak | 330 | 7 | 6 | 50 | 470 |
| Healthy Choice Beef Tip Francais | 280 | 5 | 4 | 30 | 520 |
| Healthy Choice Yankee Roast | 290 | 7 | 4 | 55 | 460 |
| Healthy Choice Mesquite Beef with Barbecue Sauce | 320 | 9 | 5 | 55 | 490 |
| Lean Cuisine Beef Pot Roast | 210 | 7 | 3 | 40 | 570 |
| Lean Cuisine Macaroni and Beef | 270 | 5 | 4 | 25 | 590 |

| Meal | Calories | Fat (gm) | Fiber (gm) | Choles-terol (mg) | Sodium (mg) |
|---|---|---|---|---|---|
| *Beef (continued)* | | | | | |
| Smart Ones Swedish Meatballs | 300 | 10 | 2 | 50 | 510 |
| Smart Ones Lasagna with Meat Sauce | 240 | 2 | 4 | 10 | 520 |
| *Pasta and Cheese* | | | | | |
| Healthy Choice Macaroni and Cheese | 320 | 7 | 4 | 25 | 580 |
| Healthy Choice Pasta Shells Marinara | 390 | 8 | 5 | 40 | 390 |
| Lean Cuisine Fettucini Primavera | 270 | 7 | 4 | 15 | 580 |
| Lean Cuisine Cheese Ravioli | 270 | 7 | 5 | 45 | 580 |
| Smart Ones Fettucini Alfredo | 230 | 6 | 3 | 20 | 540 |
| *Ethnic* | | | | | |
| Budget Gourmet Chinese Style Vegetables and White Chicken in Sauce with Rice | 250 | 7 | 3 | 15 | 640 |
| Budget Gourmet Spicy Szechwan Style Vegetables and White Chicken in Sauce with Noodles | 290 | 9 | 3 | 15 | 890 |
| Healthy Choice Chicken Teriyaki | 270 | 6 | 3 | 45 | 600 |
| Lean Cuisine Oriental Beef | 220 | 5 | 2 | 30 | 590 |
| Smart Ones Chicken Chow Mein | 200 | 2 | 3 | 25 | 570 |

*Source:* Manufacturers' Food Labels

these dinners from pasta primavera to herb roasted chicken are downright delicious.

Frozen dinners aren't just for dinners. Anytime is the right time. A microwavable frozen meal makes a great lunch. Stock up your work place freezer with a selection of frozen entrées. When the only thing to eat is a vending machine candy bar, that frozen meal alternative is a heart saver. Depending on your taste, frozen meals can be eaten for breakfast, too. I personally like pasta in the a.m. (hey, I'm Italian!), and with a piece of fruit, I'm set for the morning.

Years ago, frozen dinners typically meant oodles of un-wanted fat and sodium with little in the way of fiber and other heart-healthy nutrients. Today's frozen dinners are different. You can easily find good tasting, low fat, low sodium frozen meals that also pack some fiber, vitamins, and minerals. Selecting a frozen dinner or entrée that fits into your Simple Six Eating Plan is a snap. Use these five quick-check guidelines when navigating the frozen food aisle. You might be surprised at how many new and exciting frozen entrées there are in the frozen food case.

1. *Calorie and fat budget—Shoot for 300 to 400 calories and 10 to 13 grams of fat per meal.* Keep calorie and fat counts at or below these target ranges. Many frozen meals have over 1000 calories and 30 grams of fat. Look for those that are moderate in calories and less than 30 percent fat calories.

2. *Sodium ceiling—600 milligrams.* Frozen meals are notoriously high in sodium. If you're watching high blood pressure, check the sodium content on the label. You can always spice up your meal with herbs, fresh garlic, hot sauce, and other low-sodium seasonings.

3. *Cholesterol limit—less than 150 milligrams.* Frozen meals that in-clude meats, eggs, and cheese also come with cholesterol. Lower-fat entrées typically are not high in cholesterol, and vegetarian meals have none as long as milk, egg, or cheese are not ingredients.

4. *Fiber goal—five or more grams per meal.* Select frozen meals that include vegetables, whole-grain side dishes, and fruit for a dose of fiber. Foods made with refined ingredients such as plain pasta or those without added vegetables have next to nothing in the way of fiber.

5. *Think variety.* Try an array of frozen dinners and entrées—from standards such as Salisbury steak to Szechwan chicken. Branching out not only exposes you to new flavors, but you also get a variety of nutrients.

### Meal Add-ons

Many frozen meals come with a half cup of vegetables or less and may even skip the fruit altogether. You can easily boost the fiber, vitamins, and minerals of your favorite frozen meal with these side-dish suggestions:

- Add on to the frozen meal by placing several baby carrots or broccoli florets in the microwave during cooking.
- Microwave a baked potato and top with cooked broccoli or fresh chopped tomato.
- Slice fresh fruit (berries, oranges, apples, mangoes) and use as topping on nonfat vanilla yogurt.
- Toss a green salad with garbanzo or kidney beans and then dress with vinaigrette dressing.
- Toast whole-grain bread and spread with nonfat ricotta cheese.

# Garlic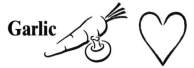

Good at warding off vampires? Maybe. Good at warding off heart disease? Definitely! This pungent member of the onion family contains compounds called *thioallyls* that research shows help dramatically lower blood cholesterol levels. These compounds also keep blood cells from clumping in arteries, thereby diverting a heart attack. These thioallyls may also be effective in lowering blood pressure. One of these compounds, called *allicin,* is released when a clove of raw garlic is crushed. Allicin not only gives garlic its characteristic smell, but also works wonders at unclogging arteries. Cooking garlic causes yet another heart-healthy compound to form, called *ajoene*, which acts a bit like aspirin and keeps the blood from clotting.

A large number of research studies show that garlic, either fresh, powdered, or extract, is effective in lowering blood cholesterol levels. In one study from the Brown University of Medicine and Memorial Hospital of Rhode Island, researchers gave men with already risky levels of LDLs garlic extract in pill form. The study participants also ate a low-fat diet.

After six months of garlic pills, researchers sampled blood cholesterol levels in the men. Blood cholesterol levels dropped significantly compared to a group of men eating the same low-fat diet and taking a placebo pill. Garlic pills also lowered LDL levels and nudged blood pressure down a few notches. Besides tasting a touch of garlic in their mouths, none of the study participants had any intestinal trouble (common with eating raw garlic).

How much garlic does the trick? A clove a day keeps the doctor away (or take at least the equivalent in powder or pill form). Should you use fresh, powdered, aged garlic extract or other types of garlic pills? According to researchers, get garlic into your diet any way you can. While it's true that raw garlic has more of the cholesterol-lowering allicin than cooked, cooked garlic has other benefits such as keeping the blood thin. Garlic pills and tablets vary in the amount of active ingredients they contain. Generally, those that are not cooked or heat treated will have more allicin.

Garlic powder available in the spice aisle at your local grocery store is one of the least expensive ways to get cholesterol-lowering allicin into your diet. Garlic powder can be added to foods during cooking or sprinkled into salads and other fresh foods. Give garlic powder a try, especially if you like fresh garlic, but it doesn't like you.

Fresh garlic, crushed or chopped, can be added to virtually anything. When selecting garlic in the produce aisle, look for firm, compact bulbs without any green sprouts coming out of the ends (a sign that it's old). You can also purchase ready-to-use crushed garlic in jars. Check the label as oil is often added. But since a teaspoon or two of garlic is used in cooking (unless you want to wake up your neighbors with your breath), this extra oil is not worth the worry. One of my favorite ways to enjoy garlic is baking whole bulbs and then spreading soft, creamy garlic on toasted sourdough bread.

## *Baked Garlic*

4 garlic heads

1 tbsp. olive oil

Using a sharp knife, cut off the tops (about a half inch) of each garlic head. Place in a glass baking dish with a half-inch of water. Drizzle the oil evenly over the tops and cover the baking dish with a lid or foil. Bake in a 350-degree oven for 40 minutes; remove the lid and bake another 10 minutes until soft. Spread on toasted sourdough bread with a sprinkle of grated Parmesan cheese. Serves four.

| **Nutrition Facts** | |
| :--- | ---: |
| Baked Garlic | |
| Serving Size 1 garlic head | |
| **Amount per Serving** | |
| Calories 119      33 Calories from fat | |
| | % Daily Value |
| Total Fat 4g | 6% |
| Saturated Fat <1g | 3% |
| Cholesterol 0mg | 0% |
| Sodium 10mg | 0% |
| Total Carbohydrate 20g | 7% |
| Dietary Fiber 1g | 4% |
| Protein 4g | |
| Vitamin A 0%   •   Vitamin C 31% | |
| Calcium 11%   •   Iron 6% | |
| •   Vitamin $B_6$ 37% | |

# Ginger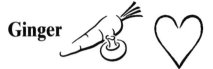

Since 600 B.C., this zippy-tasting spice has been used by the Chinese. During the Middle Ages, ginger became an indispensable flavoring agent for sauce recipes (popular to drown out the bad taste of often spoiled meat; refrigeration was still 2500 years away). Ginger is also used for medicinal purposes. This underground stem known as a rhizome is steeped in hot water to make a therapeutic tea. In India, for example, ginger tea is used to treat digestive problems and cold symptoms. But ginger may do more than unstuff your nose. Research suggests ginger may act much like aspirin and keep the blood from clotting.

Scientists from India and Denmark gave patients who already had heart disease a single dose of two teaspoons of powdered ginger. The participants' blood was then sampled and tested for its degree of "stickiness," an indication of how easily the blood would clot. The ginger dose significantly reduced the ability of the blood to clot, much the same way aspirin does.

Before you swallow two teaspoons of ginger, know this would pack quite a punch to your taste buds. It's not clear how much fresh ginger would have the same benefit. Until there's more research, try adding fresh or dry ginger to your favorite recipes. Fresh grated ginger works well in stir-fries, cold salads, and even smoothies. (Try my Ginger & Gold Salad recipe.) When buying ginger, select dense roots without shriveled skin or discolored ends. Ginger keeps for several weeks in the refrigerator when wrapped in a moist paper towel and placed in a plastic bag.

### *Ginger & Gold Salad*

3 cups cooked (buckwheat) soban noodles (sold in the Asian food section)

1 yellow pepper, seeded and chopped into small pieces

2 tsp. grated fresh ginger

1 yellow tomato, chopped

1/2 cup nori, slivered (sold in Asian food section)

1/2 shredded Chinese cabbage

Combine all of the above ingredients in a large salad bowl. Toss lightly with the dressing and refrigerate one hour before serving. Serves six.

*Dressing:* 1/4 cup rice vinegar, 2 tablespoons sesame oil, 1 teaspoon sesame seeds, 1 teaspoon crushed garlic, 2 tablespoons fish sauce (optional; sold in Asian food section).

| Nutrition Facts | |
| --- | --- |
| Ginger & Gold Salad | |
| Serving Size 1/6 recipe | |
| **Amount per Serving** | |
| Calories 168    45 Calories from fat | |
| | % Daily Value |
| Total Fat 5g | 8% |
| Saturated Fat <1g | 4% |
| Cholesterol 0mg | 0% |
| Sodium 70mg | 3% |
| Total Carbohydrate 26g | 9% |
| Dietary Fiber 2g | 7% |
| Protein 5g | |
| Vitamin A 17%  •  Vitamin C 70% | |
| Calcium 2%  •  Iron 3% | |
| •  Vitamin E 20% | |

# Grapefruit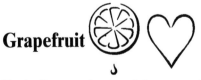

Typically served at breakfast, grapefruit is a nutritional bargain for heart health. One-half of a medium-sized grapefruit has only 40 calories and loads of goodies that protect your heart like a hefty dose of vitamin C, folic acid, and potassium. And if you like the ruby red grapefruit, more good news. Lycopene, which gives grapefruit its red color, helps protect the LDL from oxidizing and damaging artery walls. Grapefruit also contains a special fiber called *pectin*. In your intestinal tract, pectin grabs onto cholesterol and keeps it from getting into your system and clogging your arteries.

Grapefruit fiber, according to research studies, can really put a damper on cholesterol levels. In one investigation, a group of men and women, who had cholesterol levels in the danger zone, were given a five-gram dose of grapefruit pectin three times a day with meals. During the four weeks they were on the supplement, no other changes were made in the participants' diets. That is, they were not eating a low-fat diet or making any effort to lower their blood cholesterol levels.

At the end of the month-long treatment, the researchers discovered some staggering news: Blood cholesterol levels dropped over seven percent and LDL, the "bad" carrier of cholesterol, fell a whopping 11 percent. The researchers were impressed with these results not only because the fiber was given for just four weeks, but also, the subjects weren't exactly making an effort with their diets to lower cholesterol levels.

The amount of pectin taken daily by these participants would require eating at least three to four whole grapefruits daily. This may seem excessive, but including grapefruit on a regular basis as part of your Simple Six Eating Plan will help you keep heart disease at bay. Instead of sectioning a grapefruit half, just peel away the outer skin and eat like an orange. This way you get more of the pectin fiber.

Select grapefruit that is firm and slightly springy to the touch. They store well for a few weeks in the refrigerator, but if opened use within a day or two. In addition to starting off your day with a grapefruit half, peel and add the sections to green salads, fruit salads, and smoothies. My Grapefruit-Shrimp Salad recipe may have some "different" ingredients, but I'm sure you'll find it tasty.

(Note for those of you on medications: Grapefruit contains a special phytochemical called *naringenin* which can change the effectiveness of drugs you may be taking for hypertension, as well as other drugs. Naringenin slows the liver's breakdown of drugs. Studies show that drinking grapefruit juice with high blood pressure medication boosts the drug's action. Check with your physician before combining your medications with grapefruit or grapefruit juice.)

## *Grapefruit-Shrimp Salad*

4 large grapefruit, peeled and chopped into chunks the size of a quarter

1/2 red onion, sliced into strips

8 oz. of precooked shrimp (if using frozen, thaw first)

2 tbsp. raspberry vinaigrette

1/4 cup chopped coriander

fresh ground pepper to taste (optional)

In a bowl, toss all the ingredients making sure the vinaigrette is evenly distributed. Chill for 1 hour. Serves four.

| **Nutrition Facts** | |
| --- | --- |
| Grapefruit-Shrimp Salad | |
| Serving Size 1/4 recipe | |
| Amount per Serving | |
| Calories 175 | 54 Calories from fat |
| | % Daily Value |
| Total Fat 5g | 8% |
| Saturated Fat 1g | 5% |
| Cholesterol 86mg | 29% |
| Sodium 85mg | 4% |
| Total Carbohydrate 21g | 7% |
| Dietary Fiber 3g | 14% |
| Protein 13g | |
| Vitamin A 11% • Vitamin C 160% | |
| Calcium 6% • Iron 10% | |

## Grapes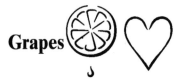

We all can picture a cluster of deep red grapes, sweetened by the sun. Beautiful, yes; but when you look at grapes' nutritional profile, it's rather unremarkable. A cup of table grapes supply about 100 calories and very modest amounts of fiber, vitamin C, and other nutrients except potassium with about eight percent of daily needs in one serving. But beauty is more than skin deep. The fact is, grapes' heart-saving qualities are actually found in the grape skins and seeds. Several flavonoids, a type of phytochemical found in fruits and some vegetables, abound in grapes. And it's the flavonoids that make their way from grape skins into red wine giving this beverage its heart-healthy reputation.

A wide range of research studies have shown that the grape flavonoids help fight heart disease by lowering blood cholesterol levels. Also, one flavonoid in particular, called *resveratrol*, found in fresh grapes, grape juice, grape jelly, and red wine, has been shown to help protect the bad carrier of cholesterol, LDL, from damaging artery walls. Keeping LDLs from going "bad" or oxidizing, means heart disease is thwarted. By the way, white wine has very little resveratrol because grape skins are removed early in the fermenting process of white wine (that's why white wine is clear or colorless. For more on wine see page 290.)

Both green and red grape varieties contain flavonoids. Since grapes are available year round (peak season June through November), try different types, with and without seeds, so your heart can experience an array of flavonoids. Look for grapes in your produce section that are in compact clusters with good color. Since grapes do not ripen after they are picked, don't expect them to get any sweeter in your kitchen.

Grapes add vibrant color and a sweet taste to fruit salads as well as green salads. You can also use grapes in your favorite stuffing recipe for turkey or chicken. Fresh grapes add needed moisture and a wonderful taste, along with heart-healthy flavonoids, to your holiday feast. Try out my salad recipe.

## *Grape-Tofu Curry Salad*

1 cup green and red grapes, sliced in half

1 cup firm tofu, cut into half-inch cubes

1 cup cooked chicken, cubed (or omit chicken and use two cups tofu total)

1/4 cup fat-free ranch dressing

1/2 cup nonfat plain yogurt

3/4 tsp. curry powder

fresh ground pepper to taste

3/4 cup celery, chopped

3/4 cup water chestnuts, sliced

chopped scallions for garnish

Mix dressing, yogurt, and spices together in a bowl. Add tofu (chicken), celery, and water chestnuts, stir well and cover. Refrigerate one hour. Serve over lettuce and garnish with scallions. Makes four servings.

| **Nutrition Facts** | |
|---|---|
| Grape-Tofu Curry Salad | |
| Serving Size 1 1/4 cup | |
| Amount per Serving | |
| Calories 227     75 Calories from fat | |
| | % Daily Value |
| Total Fat 8g | 13% |
| Saturated Fat 1g | 6% |
| Cholesterol 37mg | 12% |
| Sodium 216mg | 9% |
| Total Carbohydrate 18g | 6% |
| Dietary Fiber 3g | 10% |
| Protein 21g | |
| Vitamin A 2%   •   Vitamin C 11% | |
| Calcium 14%   •   Iron 25% | |

# Guava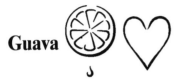

A tropical delight that your heart thanks you for, guava comes packed with three power players to help fight heart disease and hypertension—vitamin C, potassium, and fiber. A medium-sized guava (about three inches in diameter) supplies a whopping 275 percent of vitamin C needs, a load of potassium, and 20 percent of your fiber needs all in a mere 45 calories. These three heart savers work together and according to research studies, eating guavas daily lowers cholesterol and blood pressure.

In one study, scientists from the Heart Research Laboratory in Moradabad in India gathered over 100 subjects with hypertension, including some who had dangerous cholesterol levels. Half of the participants were asked to eat about four to seven guavas daily for 12 weeks while the other group was "business as usual," making no changes to their diets. This 12-week period of eating guava greatly boosted their intake of vitamin C, potassium, and fiber. And with great results. Cholesterol levels fell a hefty 10 percent which translates to a 20 percent reduction in heart-disease risk. HDL, the cholesterol good guy, went up and blood pressure fell. What more could you ask for in a fruit?

Researchers and others have noted that it is the magical combination of vitamin C, potassium, and fiber in guava that gives it its miraculous abilities. Vitamin C is a powerful antioxidant that may help LDLs from becoming oxidized and injuring artery walls; potassium puts a damper on blood pressure as it helps balance sodium; and the fiber in guava is a cholesterol "snatcher." Water-soluble fiber, the type in guava, scoops up cholesterol in the intestinal tract preventing it from getting inside the body to do any damage.

It sounds as though guavas should make an appearance in your diet. Select fruit without blemishes or broken skin. They ripen well in a fruit bowl and will be slightly soft to the touch with a notable tropical fragrance when ripe. Guava's fleshy inside is usually yellow or even pinkish and wonderfully sweet. You can add guavas to smoothies and fruit salads; or top your morning cereal or a cup of nonfat vanilla yogurt with diced ripe guavas. Guavas can be mashed into a puree and heated for a delicious sauce to top grilled fish or chicken.

# Herbs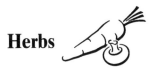

A look at the textbook definition of herbs gives you the idea that these aromatic leaves, stems and flowers of certain edible plants (such as basil, dill, and mint) merely serve as flavoring agents. Hardly. Herbs protect your heart and ward off high blood pressure in a way that's unlike most super-foods. It's true that by themselves, herbs have little to offer nutritionally since they are typically used in small amounts.

But herbs' heart-saving qualities stem from modifying what you *would have* put in your food. Used to enhance foods' natural flavors, herbs can easily take the place of heart-stopping ingredients such as added fat and salt. This means, for example, that instead of a traditionally high-fat cream sauce that you would have poured over grilled fish, you can substitute fresh herbs as a flavorful and healthful alternative.

A variety of herbs is sold fresh in your local supermarket. You can also find dried herbs in the spice section. Go for the fresh when given a choice since the flavor of fresh herbs outshines the dried version. Fresh herbs keep about a week in the refrigerator when kept in a plastic bag with a slightly moist paper towel around their base. This method keeps herbs from wilting or getting slimy, a sign of bacterial contamination.

While the flavor of dried herbs is not always as distinctive as fresh, they are certainly more convenient. When kept in an airtight container, dried herbs can be kept for a year or more. In most recipes you can interchange fresh and dried herbs. As a general rule, about one-third to one-half teaspoon of dried herbs is equivalent to one tablespoon of fresh.

Herbs can be used in virtually any dish from salads and soups to side dishes and entrées to desserts and beverages. Knowing what herbs go well with certain foods and combinations of

# Make a Match

---

Common herbs and foods that work well together.

---

**Anise:** some vegetables like carrots and spinach, eggs, fish, fruit, poultry, and pork; also delicious in baked goods such as coffee cakes, cookies, and fruit cobblers.

**Basil:** a favorite in tomato dishes, most other vegetables, beef, soups, eggs, fish, lamb, pasta, poultry, potatoes, rice, veal.

**Bay Leaf:** beef, chicken, tomatoes, veal, meat marinades, casseroles.

**Chives:** chicken, corn, many vegetables such as asparagus and tomatoes, fish, potatoes, veal.

**Cinnamon:** baked breads, muffins, and cookies; chicken, fruit, lamb.

**Coriander:** most vegetables, beef, chicken, eggs, fish, fruit salsas, lamb, rice, tomatoes.

**Cumin:** beef, chicken, lamb, many vegetables such as carrots and cauliflower.

**Dill:** chicken, eggs, vegetables such as squash and tomatoes, fish, lamb, potatoes.

**Marjoram:** beef, chicken, fish, turkey, veal, vegetables including broccoli and tomatoes, eggs.

**Mint:** vegetables including green beans and carrots, fruit, beverages such as brewed teas, lamb, veal.

**Oregano:** beef, chicken, eggplant, eggs, fish, mushrooms, pork, potatoes, squash, tomatoes, turkey.

**Parsley:** most vegetables, beef, chicken, eggs, fish, lamb, tomatoes, veal.

**Rosemary:** beef, chicken, eggs, fish, fruit, pork, potatoes, spinach, turkey, veal.

**Saffron:** eggs, fish, lamb, rice.

**Sage:** vegetables including green beans, squash, and tomatoes; beef, chicken, eggs, fish, potatoes, turkey, veal.

**Tarragon:** beef, chicken, eggs, fish, lamb, pork, potatoes, many vegetables including carrots and tomatoes.

**Thyme:** beef, chicken, eggs, fish, lamb, turkey, veal, many vegetables including mushrooms and tomatoes.

foods simply takes some experimenting. If you've never really given herbs a try, get started with my "Make a Match" herb listing. This listing gives you an idea what foods go best with various herbs.

# Hot Peppers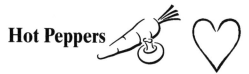

From mild to fiery hot, you've got to love those peppers. In fact, some people gobble down scorching hot peppers, suffering watery eyes, runny noses, and burning mouths, only to go back for more. Many scientists believe that hot-pepper addicts may be just that, addicted to the pain or to the brain chemicals released in response to the mouth fire. But with pain there is pleasure, at least for your heart. Hot peppers protect your heart with almost 200 percent of vitamin C needs per serving and special phytochemicals called *flavonoids.*

Hot peppers contain a variety of flavonoids and one of those, *capsaicin,* is actually responsible for the fiery taste. Another flavonoid, called *quercetin,* also found in onions and red wine, has been shown to help ward off heart disease. When put to the test, quercetin keeps LDLs, the bad cholesterol, from becoming a hazard to artery walls. Quercetin's protecting action explains why people who consume diets rich in this flavonoid have a significantly lower risk for heart disease. Along with the vitamin C that also acts like quercetin, hot peppers make a "hot" addition to your Simple Six Eating Plan.

With the variety of hot peppers, you can easily suit your taste for spicy. Check out my "Hot Lover's Guide to Peppers" and experiment with different hot peppers in a variety of dishes. Select peppers that have smooth skin without soft or sunken spots. Peppers store well in the refrigerator if kept free of excessive moisture which can cause spoilage.

Hot peppers go in just about any dish as long as you like it hot (well, almost any dish—as a topping for ice cream would sure keep me away). Salsa made from fresh tomatoes, garlic, onions,

## Hot Lover's Guide to Peppers

Here's a rundown on some of the many varieties of hot
or chili peppers available.

*Anaheim or New Mexican chili:*  Mild, long green chilies; great in casseroles, mixed with eggs, and in mild salsas.

*Cayenne:*  Used in its dried form, usually powdered, cayenne is very hot. A favorite in Cajun dishes.

*Habanero:*  Small, pumpkin-looking green or red chili that is as hot as you can get. Best used by hot pepper aficionados.

*Jalapeño:*  Hot, small green chili that is the most popular hot pepper around. Works well in burritos, salsas, nachos, eggs, casseroles, and just about everything—even on top of pizza.

*Serrano:*  Hot, small green chilies that are best used fresh in salsas.

*Yellow wax:*  Hot, yellow chili that adds manageable fire to soups, stews, and salsas.

and hot peppers (see my recipe) is a no-fat heart-saving dip for veggie sticks or chips (low-fat, of course). Try hot peppers in stir-fries, burritos, stews, soups, and even fresh green salads for a kick. Remember, if you ever go overboard on the hot peppers, you can cool your mouth off with a piece of bread or a swallow of milk. Quenching the fire with water will only spread it!

### *Hot and Heart-Healthy Salsa*

2 med. tomatoes, chopped

2 cloves of garlic, crushed

1 med. jalapeño, chopped (to avoid contact with skin use a food processor). Try other peppers to suit taste.

1/2 red onion, chopped

1/4 cup chopped cilantro

Mix all ingredients together in a bowl and it's ready for dipping. Fresh cut-up vegetables, wedges of whole-wheat pita bread, or soft tortilla as well as chips make great dipping tools. Or use salsa to top tacos, egg dishes, baked potatoes, or anything you wish.

| Nutrition Facts | |
| :--- | ---: |
| Hot and Heart-Healthy Salsa | |
| Serving Size 1/4 cup | |
| **Amount per Serving** | |
| Calories 33        0 Calories from fat | |
| | **% Daily Value** |
| Total Fat 0g | 0% |
| Saturated Fat 0g | 0% |
| Cholesterol 0mg | 0% |
| Sodium 0mg | 0% |
| Total Carbohydrate 6g | 2% |
| Dietary Fiber 2g | 7% |
| Protein 1g | |
| Vitamin A 20%  •  Vitamin C 70% | |
| Calcium 2%      •  Iron 2% | |

# Ice Cream

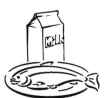

From the moment a spoonful of creamy, sinfully-rich premium ice cream hits your mouth, you know there's no way this delight could ever be good for you. A friend of mine jokes that you may as well open up his heart and stuff the ice cream right in because he knows "it's killing me but I love the stuff." And who doesn't? We spend an estimated $3 billion yearly on ice cream with no signs of slowing this indulgence. And a heart-stopping indulgence it is.

In an extreme case of ice-cream madness, a 54-year-old British man admitted to eating three to sometimes six quarts daily over a three-month period. As a result, his cholesterol levels were literally off the charts, not to mention he was taking in over 500 grams of fat daily! Once he curtailed his ice cream intake, his blood cholesterol levels dropped dramatically. While three quarts may exceed your daily quota, how does an ice-cream lover keep heart disease and hypertension in check without giving up you know what?

For starters, ice cream's nutritional stats would easily scare any artery. A half-cup serving (who eats only half a cup?) of full-fat ice cream (often called super-premium with 16 percent butterfat) has over 180 calories and a whopping 16 grams of fat, mostly artery-clogging saturated fat. Premium brands with 14 percent butterfat aren't much better. And regular ice cream, your basic store-brand variety with 12 percent butterfat has over 150 calories and nine grams of fat. But don't despair; great tasting lower-fat versions of ice cream populate the frozen foods section waiting for your taste buds' approval.

Low-fat ice cream with only three grams of fat per half cup tastes like the real McCoy, minus much of the artery-choking saturated fat. And fat-free ice cream, a decent tasting substitute, has just a speck of fat. But check the labels for "reduced" fat and "light" ice creams which are required to have 25 percent and 33 percent less fat, respectively, than the standard. Also, frozen

## What's the Scoop

Calories and fat facts on ice cream and frozen yogurt.

| 1/2 Cup Serving | Calories | Fat (grams) | Saturated Fat (grams) |
|---|---|---|---|
| Ben & Jerry's | 250 | 14 | 9 |
| Häagen-Dazs | 310 | 23 | 11 |
| Dryer's | 170 | 10 | 5 |
| Light ice cream, vanilla | 120 | 4.5 | 3 |
| Low-fat ice cream, vanilla | 170 | 2.5 | 1.5 |
| Fat-free ice cream, vanilla | 100 | 0 | 0 |
| Frozen yogurt, vanilla | 100 | 2.5 | 1.5 |
| Low-fat frozen yogurt, vanilla | 100 | 2.5 | 1.5 |
| Fat-free frozen yogurt, vanilla | 90 | 0 | 0 |

*Source:* Manufacturers' Food Labels

yogurt is not necessarily lower in fat than reduced-fat or low-fat ice cream. Some frozen yogurts contain as much fat as regular 12 percent butterfat ice cream. Check out the fat facts on frozen treats in the "What's the Scoop" chart.

Keep in mind that all the low-fat and sans fat ice creams still come with a dose of calories (mostly from sugar). This means that loading your bowl with a hefty serving of fat-free ice cream can easily contribute to weight gain even though it's fat-free. As with other "extra" foods, use moderation when dishing up your favorite frozen treat. Ice cream, preferably fat-free, can easily fit into your Simple Six Eating Plan, just not three quarts daily!

# Kale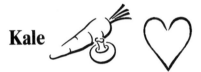

Kale is a green leafy vegetable; and a green leafy vegetable is a leaf. Your mother probably told you to eat your green leafy vegetables. But kale, and the others (arugula, endive, and more) look more like rabbit food than anything else you might eat. Of course, mom was right. Green leafy veggies like kale should be a staple in your diet to ward off heart disease and hypertension.

Kale is loaded with carotenes called *lutein* and *zeaxanthin* (a mouthful to say) that act as antioxidants protecting you from heart disease. Greens like kale are also a great source of the minerals magnesium, calcium and potassium for lowering high blood pressure. There's more: Greens also supply folate, the B vitamin that helps lower levels of the blood factor homocysteine that damages artery walls. And kale, along with many other greens, packs a good dose of vitamin C, another antioxidant that fends off heart disease.

A host of research studies shows that people who skimp on greens and other carotene-rich foods have higher death rates from heart disease and stroke. The same is true for people who fall short on meeting their vitamin C needs. The antioxidants— carotenes and vitamin C—are known to protect the bad carrier of cholesterol, LDLs, from becoming hazardous to artery walls causing fatty plaque buildup.

# Guide to Greens

Green leafy vegetables are more than a tossed salad. From arugala to watercress, greens come in a variety of shapes and flavors, but for the most part, green leafy veggies are leaves, and . . . green. Here's a quick rundown on greens available at your local supermarket.

**Arugula:** Distinctive peppery flavor, dandelion-shaped leaves of medium green; adds sharp zing to salads, soups, or omelets.

**Basil:** Deep green small leaves, aromatic and strong flavor; use fresh in pasta and salads, and of course, great mixed with crushed garlic as pesto.

**Beet greens:** Cabbage-like flavor, dark-green rough leaves with red stalk; best in soups or use sparingly as part of a green salad mix.

**Bok choy:** Mild cabbage flavor, celery-like stalks with deep green leaf, from the cruciferous vegetable family; a stir-fry staple (see recipe), or add to soups.

**Chicory greens (curly endive):** Slightly bitter or tart taste, frilly-looking medium green leaves; use in salads as part of a mix, or add to hearty stews for extra flavor.

**Chinese cabbage:** Bumpy lighter green leaves, mild flavor; use like regular cabbage in coleslaw or cold chicken salad, also great in soup.

**Collard greens:** Big deep green leaves, stronger cabbage flavor; use as vegetable side dish, or in stir-fries, soups, and stews.

**Dandelion greens:** Spiked shaped leaves, bitter flavor, medium-green; great in salads or served wilted over fish.

**Endive:** Long, smooth leaves (sometimes very pale color), bitter but lively flavor; good in salads.

**Kale:** Bold green leaves with rippled edges, cabbage-like flavor; best steamed as side dish, or add chopped to stir-fries, soups, or stews.

**Mustard greens:** Deep green leaves with curled edges, mild peppery taste; use in soups, stews, or sparingly in salads.

**Purslane:** Smaller clover-shaped leaves, tart taste; use in salads, in sandwiches, or steamed slightly as a side dish.

**Radichio:** Striking red cabbage-like leaf, mild to strong cabbage flavor; a salad standout or use for color and taste in stir-fries.

**Romaine lettuce:** Large ruffled green leaves (pale at their base), mild flavor; great as a salad or wilted and served with entrée.

**Spinach:** Deep green oval-shaped leaves, mildly spicy or tart taste; excellent as a salad, steam for a side dish, or add to stir-fries, soups, quiche, and casseroles.

**Swiss chard:** Large glossy green leaves, strong flavor; steam as a side dish, great as a pasta filling mixed with low-fat cheese, or mix in salads.

**Turnip greens:** Musty green leaves, cabbage flavor; great steamed as a side dish, or added to soups and stews, or use sparingly in salads.

**Watercress:** Small deep green leaves, spicy flavor; use in salads and sandwich mixes.

If you're like many people though, the only green leafy vegetable you eat regularly is iceberg lettuce, which unfortunately, doesn't have the same heart-saving attributes of other leafy greens. It's time to turn over a new leaf, and a green one at that. Next time you're in the produce aisle, select a new green leafy vegetable. Check out the "Guide to Greens" for a primer on the many different types of greens and their uses. I also include my speedy recipe for using greens in ready-made soup. (Also, see Spinach on page 255 for more about greens including storing information and recipes.)

### Lentil Soup à la Greens

2 cans lentil soup

1 cup chopped kale and mustard greens

1 clove crushed garlic

1/4 tsp. ground cumin

Heat soup with garlic and cumin until simmering. Add greens and cook a few minutes until fully wilted. Serves four.

| **Nutrition Facts** | |
|---|---|
| Lentil Soup à la Greens | |
| Serving Size 1/4 recipe | |
| Amount per Serving | |
| Calories 148        18 Calories from fat | |
| | % Daily Value |
| Total Fat 2g | 3% |
| Saturated Fat 0g | 0% |
| Cholesterol 0mg | 0% |
| Sodium 750mg | 30% |
| Total Carbohydrate 24g | 8% |
| Dietary Fiber 8g | 32% |
| Protein 10g | |
| Vitamin A 28%  •  Vitamin C 25% | |
| Calcium 6%  •  Iron 22% | |

# Kiwifruit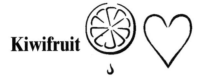

They are soft and fuzzy brown on the outside, but packed with hard-hitting nutrition on the inside. Kiwifruit's bright green, tart-tasting flesh is loaded with an array of heart-healthy vitamins and minerals. A recent study from the Department of Food Science at Rutgers University in New Jersey compared kiwifruit to 24 other frequently eaten fruits including apples, bananas, and oranges, and found kiwi to be the most nutrient dense fruit. So ounce for ounce, kiwifruit comes packed with the most vitamin and mineral nutrition.

On top of the list is vitamin C, a powerful antioxidant that keeps the bad guy, LDL cholesterol, from damaging artery walls. One medium-sized kiwi has over 130 percent of daily vitamin C needs. Kiwi also contains a dose of another notable antioxidant that is not commonly found in other fruits, vitamin E. Researchers have discovered that vitamin E actually sits on the surface of LDLs, keeping them from oxidizing and becoming hazardous to your heart.

Kiwifruit also comes equipped with three super minerals that help keep blood pressure in check—calcium, magnesium, and potassium. Several studies show that low intakes of these minerals are linked to the development of hypertension. And since few fruits supply much in the way of calcium and magnesium, kiwifruit should make a regular appearance in your fruit bowl. Besides kiwifruit's wondrous supply of vitamins and minerals, each piece provides over 10 percent of fiber needs. And the fiber in kiwifruit is the type that helps lower blood cholesterol. All said and done, kiwifruit has an amazing amount of heart-healthy goodies for only 46 calories in one medium-sized fruit.

Purchase kiwifruit either ripe (gives slightly to pressure), or firm and let it ripen at home in a fruit bowl or paper bag. Avoid fruit that has any broken marks or deep blemishes. Kiwifruit out-lasts most other fruits; it keeps for weeks in your refrigerator. How to eat a kiwi? If you're after lots of fiber, just rinse it off and bite right into that fuzzy brown skin. Or you can cut a kiwifruit in half and spoon out the fruit much like you would eat a grapefruit. Or better yet, you can peel off the brown skin and slice or dice kiwifruit.

Use kiwifruit to top off your cereal, yogurt, or waffles. Or add some kiwi-green color to smoothies, pasta, and fruit salads. You can also use sliced kiwi the same way as sliced tomatoes, such as in sandwiches or atop crackers as an appetizer. One of my favorite ways to eat kiwifruit is in a zesty fruit salsa that compliments grilled fish, chicken, or lean beef. Try out my recipe. This salsa also goes great with black beans and rice.

### Sassy Fruit Salsa

2 med. kiwifruit, peeled and diced

1 small red onion (or 1/2 large one), finely chopped

1 red bell pepper, seeded and chopped

1 yellow or orange bell pepper, seeded and chopped

1/3 cup fresh cilantro, finely chopped

1 clove garlic, crushed or finely chopped

1/4 tsp. red pepper flakes

2 tbsp. pineapple juice or juice from one lemon

**Nutrition Facts**
Sassy Fruit Salsa
Serving Size 1/6 recipe

| Amount per Serving | |
|---|---|
| Calories 30 | 0 Calories from fat |

| | % Daily Value |
|---|---|
| Total Fat 0g | 0% |
| Saturated Fat 0g | 0% |
| Cholesterol 0mg | 0% |
| Sodium 0mg | 0% |
| Total Carbohydrate 7g | 2% |
| Dietary Fiber 2g | 6% |
| Protein 1g | |

Vitamin A 10% • Vitamin C 100%
Calcium <2% • Iron 2%

Combine all ingredients in a bowl being sure pepper flakes are distributed evenly in the mixture. Chill before serving. Makes six servings.

# Lemons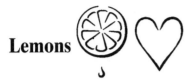

The smell of fresh lemons invigorates; it even makes some people salivate. The aroma is so appealing that we purchase lemon scented furniture polish and cleaners. For you lemon lovers, here's some good news: The substance that makes a lemon smell like a lemon is good for your heart. *Limonene,* a type of phytochemical found primarily in the lemon peel (some in the juice), is a strong antioxidant that protects against artery damage.

## Dr. "A's" Top 10

These are my favorite ways to use lemons—juice and zest.

1. Mix lemon zest and juice into nonfat sour cream along with some parsley or chives and use to top a baked potato.

2. Put lemon juice and zest into boiling water when cooking pasta.

3. When baking fish or chicken, rub with lemon juice and zest and then sprinkle with fresh or dried herbs and bake.

4. Add lemon juice and zest to barbecue sauce for a new zing.

5. Blend lemon juice and zest in vanilla nonfat yogurt and use as a fruit dip.

6. When putting together a fresh fruit salad, toss cut fruit with lemon juice and sprinkle in lemon zest. This helps prevent browning and livens the fruits' flavor.

7. Blend nonfat mayonnaise with fresh dill, lemon juice, and zest; use for dipping artichoke leaves.

8. Sprinkle finely chopped chives, zest, and lemon juice over steamed cauliflower, carrots, or summer squash.

9. Float slices of whole lemon (rinsed well) in iced herb tea or water.

10. Add lemon juice and zest to hot tea for a soothing nightcap.

Also in the lemon peel are flavonoids that work wonders for your heart. Studies show that flavonoids help keep the blood from clumping, which can ward off heart attacks or strokes. Flavonoids also protect LDLs from corroding artery walls and may improve blood flow. Sounds great for a fruit that contains virtually no calories, is a great source of vitamin C, and makes itself at home in just about any recipe.

Shop for lemons that are firm and heavy for their size which means that they are loaded with juice. An average-sized lemon has about three tablespoons of juice. But there's more to lemons than their juice. The lemon zest or peel is loaded with limonene and flavonoids. To get the zest, take a clean, well-rinsed lemon and grate the top yellow layer off using a cheese grater. Lemon zest adds a tangy flavor to everything from beverages and desserts to sauces and baked dishes. Lemon juice along with fresh herbs makes a great substitute for salty ingredients called for in many recipes. My Caribbean Chicken recipe is packed with lemon's heart-saving goodies and is low in fat.

## *Caribbean Chicken*

4 skinless chicken breasts

zest and juice from one lemon

1/2 cup red onion, finely chopped

1 ripe mango

1 small jalapeño pepper, seeded and finely chopped

2 tbsp. honey

freshly ground pepper

dash of allspice and cinnamon

Place chicken in a glass baking dish. In a separate bowl mash the mango and combine remaining ingredients making sure to mix evenly. Spread this mixture over the chicken and cover the baking dish with foil. Bake in a 375-degree oven for 45 minutes. Uncover and broil the top until bubbly, about 10 minutes. Makes four servings.

| Nutrition Facts |  |
| --- | --- |
| Caribbean Chicken |  |
| Serving Size 1/4 recipe |  |

| Amount per Serving | |
| --- | --- |
| Calories 222      27 Calories from fat | |
|  | % Daily Value |
| Total Fat 3g | 5% |
|   Saturated Fat 1g | 5% |
| Cholesterol 73mg | 24% |
| Sodium 67mg | 3% |
| Total Carbohydrate 21g | 7% |
|   Dietary Fiber 3g | 10% |
| Protein 28g | |

| Vitamin A 37% • Vitamin C 77% |
| --- |
| Calcium 3%  •  Iron 8% |

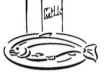

# Liver

On the one hand, liver is a nutritional powerhouse packed with an array of nutrients sure to fend off heart disease. On the other hand, liver's cholesterol content blows anyone's daily budget. My recommendation: Eat liver on occasion if you like it, but don't go out of your way to make liver a regular menu item if you are plagued by high blood cholesterol levels and your physician has cautioned you to back off on your intake.

When you dine on liver, feel good that you really are doing your heart wonders. Liver is tough to beat when it comes to the trio of B vitamins—$B_{12}$, folate, and $B_6$—that have been shown to help lower circulating levels of homocysteine, the blood factor that is directly linked to increased heart-disease risks in both men and women.

A three-ounce serving of braised liver has a staggering 3000 percent of your $B_{12}$ needs along with 90 percent of folic acid and 40 percent of your $B_6$ daily need. Considering a good one-third of the population fails to meet their requirement for these B vitamins, a serving of liver now and then makes good sense. And that's not all. Unlike most animal products, liver is a good source of vitamin C with over 30 percent of the daily dose in a serving. Along with hefty doses of the minerals iron and zinc, it's no wonder liver has its reputation as a "health" food.

You can combat some of liver's high cholesterol content—330 milligrams per serving—by serving with side dishes rich in cholesterol-busting nutrients. Prepare liver in a nonstick skillet and serve up with cooked barley, a fresh green salad tossed with peppers, walnuts, and a flax seed dressing, and topped off with baked apples for dessert.

# Mango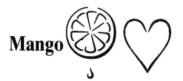

Whenever I eat a mango, thoughts of the tropics come to mind. I like to use this exotic fruit in smoothies or as a puree for topping pancakes. Despite its "paradise" image, mango is a tough player when it comes to fighting off hypertension. With a whopping 100 percent of your vitamin C needs along with plentiful amounts of potassium, fiber, and beta carotene in one mango, this fruit should be a regular addition to your daily fare.

Mango's one-two combination of vitamin C and potassium make this fruit particularly beneficial for those of you controlling high blood pressure. A variety of studies show that people who take in adequate vitamin C from fruits like mango have greater circulating levels of this vitamin which in turn has been linked to lower blood pressure. Researchers from the Medical College of Georgia found that people in their study with low circulating vitamin C levels were at risk for hypertension. Other research shows that low intake of potassium correlates strongly to hypertension risk. Bottom line: Eat mangos in your fight against hypertension.

Look for mangos in your supermarket's produce section year-round, though a bit pricey during the winter months. Select fruit that is green with freckles and has a reddish blush. When ripe, mangos give to gentle pressure. Because the mango's pit clings to the orange flesh, simply cut the fruit off into slices or chunks. Besides smoothies, add mango pieces to a fresh fruit or green salad, use as a topper for yogurt or breakfast cereal, or chop into small pieces and make a delicious fruit salsa to accompany grilled fish or chicken. Try my mango puree on top of hot cereal, pancakes, waffles, and one of my treats, as a dip for sugar cookies. Stored in an airtight container, this puree keeps about a week.

## *Mango Mash*

2 ripe mangos, peeled with pit removed

4 to 6 tbsp. thawed, frozen orange juice concentrate

dash of cinnamon

In a food processor or blender, place all the ingredients and blend. Add more orange juice concentrate if a thinner consistency is desired. Drizzle over yogurt, hot cereal, or pancakes. Makes eight servings.

| **Nutrition Facts** | |
| --- | --- |
| Mango Mash | |
| Serving Size 1/8 recipe | |
| **Amount per Serving** | |
| Calories 55          0 Calories from fat | |
| | % Daily Value |
| Total Fat 0g | 0% |
| Saturated Fat 0g | 0% |
| Cholesterol 0mg | 0% |
| Sodium 0mg | 0% |
| Total Carbohydrate 14g | 5% |
| Dietary Fiber 2g | 8% |
| Protein <1g | |
| Vitamin A 23%  •  Vitamin C 54% | |
| Calcium 1%  •  Iron 1% | |

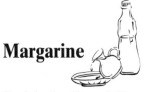

# Margarine

Back in the 40s and 50s, margarine began making inroads as a butter substitute on the tops of American's breads and potatoes, and as an ingredient in cookies and biscuits. In those days, margarine earned a good-for-you reputation as scientists began unraveling the evils attributable to butter's saturated fat and cholesterol. So in good faith, people slathered on margarine believing it was the better choice for heart health.

But margarine's image took a nose dive with the news about a phantom fat found, for the most part, only in margarine and other foods made with hydrogenated vegetable oil. During hydrogenation, which is the processing of a vegetable oil from a liquid to a solid (or semisolid), a new fat forms, called *trans* fat. Studies show that *trans* fats wreak havoc on the heart. Some medical experts suggest this phantom fat may account for an estimated 30,000 deaths yearly due to clogged arteries.

### Margarine Madness

Walk the supermarket aisle and you find scads of margarines and spreads, and even squeezable spreads, with some touting "*trans*-fat free" on their labels. Confused with all the choices? Margarine is simply an edible, spreadable fat. Like butter, stick margarine supplies 100 calories and 11 grams of fat per one-tablespoon serving. And to legally be called margarine, a product must be 80 percent fat or more by weight. The fat in margarine is strictly from vegetable oil, typically soybean, corn, safflower, and canola oil—that has been hydrogenated.

Available in tubs and squeezable bottles, margarine *spreads* contain less fat than "legal" margarine—less than 80 percent by weight (usually 60 percent) and so are lower in calories. Still, they have about 50 to 70 calories per tablespoon. Water makes up the difference in bulk, which is carefully blended in so as not to separate out from the fat. Fat-free margarine spreads and liquids available in squeeze bottles contain negligible amounts of fat, which act more like an emulsifier helping to keep water and other ingredients mixed cohesively together.

Whether sticks, tubs, or squeezables, the vegetable fat in these margarine products was once a liquid oil. The chemical process of hydrogenation chemically modifies the vegetable oils and converts them into saturated fats that, as you know, are solid at room temperature. This is why a stick of margarine or a dollop of spread holds its shape even at room temperature.

During the hydrogenation process, some of the vegetable oil gets switched around even further to form the *trans* fats. How much forms depends on the degree of hydrogenation and the type of oil used. Most servings of stick margarines contain from one to three grams of *trans* fats. In processed foods such as crackers, baked goods, and chips, hydrogenated vegetable oils (the same kind that go into margarines) are also used. Along with spreading margarine on your bread, eating chips and the like will raise your *trans* fat intake to an estimated three to twelve grams daily, a level some heart researchers consider trouble.

### Trans *Trouble*

So what's all the fuss about this new fat? In your body, scientists believe that *trans* fats do all the bad things saturated fats do to blood cholesterol levels. *Trans* fats may even be more damaging. Since very little *trans* fats occur naturally in other foods, scientists theorize we are just now seeing the artery-clogging caused by the intake of these "synthetic" fats over the past several decades. Research studies suggest that the more *trans* fats in the diet, specifically from margarine, the greater the risk of heart disease and death from heart disease.

Noted heart disease researcher Dr. Walter Willett from Harvard University studied the long-term eating habits of over 80,000 nurses. Willet found that the women with the highest intake of *trans* fats had the greatest risk for heart disease. Even those women with a high overall fat intake were at lower risk, provided their *trans* fat intake was low. Based on this research, Dr. Willett

## Stick Shift

Here's a sampling of what's in some "*trans*-fat free" spreads along with stick margarine and butter for comparison.

| Margarine or Spread (1 Tbsp.) | Calories | Fat (gm) | Saturated Fat (gm) | Trans Fat (gm) |
|---|---|---|---|---|
| Promise Ultra Fat Free, tub | 5 | 0 | 0 | 0 |
| Promise Ultra 70% Less Fat, tub | 30 | 4 | 0 | 0 |
| Promise, tub | 90 | 10 | 2 | 0 |
| Smart Beat Fat Free! Smarter Than Butter!, tub | 15 | 0 | 0 | 0 |
| Smart Beat Light Margarine, tub | 20 | 2 | 0 | 0 |
| Fleischmann's Lower Fat Margarine, tub | 40 | 5 | 0 | 0 |
| Weight Watchers Light Margarine, tub | 50 | 4 | 1 | 1 |
| I Can't Believe It's Not Butter! Light, stick | 50 | 6 | 1 | 1 |
| I Can't Believe It's Not Butter!, tub | 90 | 10 | 2 | 2 |
| Shedd's Spread Country Crock, tub | 70 | 7 | 1 | 1 |
| Land O' Lakes Country Morning Blend Light, stick or tub | 50 | 6 | 3 | 0 |
| Parkay, stick | 90 | 10 | 2 | 3 |
| Butter, stick | 100 | 11 | 7 | 0 |

*Source:* Manufacturers' Labels (in some cases, *trans* fats calculated by difference)

estimated that the risk for heart disease in these women would be cut in half if they cut back by the same amount on their *trans* fat intake. The major sources of *trans* fat for these women were margarine and other foods made with hydrogenated fat.

The trouble with *trans* fats stems from its impact on circulating cholesterol. In one study a group of 80 subjects were put on diets that provided about eight to nine percent of their total calorie intake as either *trans* fat or dairy fat (which is mostly saturated fat) for five weeks. At the end, subjects on the *trans*-fat enriched diet (about 19 grams daily) had lower levels of the cholesterol good guys, HDL, and had an increased ratio of LDL (cholesterol bad guys) to HDL compared to the dairy-fat boosted diet. All this bumps up the risk for heart disease.

### *Going Sans* Trans

Avoiding *trans* fats in the diet makes sense for your heart, but finding out where they lurk is not easy. *Trans* fats, unlike total fat and saturated fat, are not required to appear on the label. On margarines, spreads, and other butter-replacement products you can "guesstimate" the *trans* fat content by adding up the grams of saturated, monounsaturated, and polyunsaturated fat content per serving and subtracting this from the total number of fat grams per serving. The remainder should be the amount of *trans* fat in a serving.

### Designer Margarine?

The bad press about margarine's heart-wrenching *trans* fat has lead some drug companies to search for new ingredients to add in making a "designer" margarine meant to lower blood cholesterol levels. From the makers of Tylenol® comes a margarine with *sitostanol,* an extract from pine trees that lowers blood cholesterol levels. Studies show that eating three pats of margarine daily made with sitostanol lowers cholesterol levels by a dramatic 10 percent. Sold under the name of Benecol®, this margarine may help some lower dangerously high cholesterol levels.

What amount of *trans* fat is safe is not known. Until more research unfolds the exact nature of *trans* fats, it's best to try to avoid margarines with *trans* fats. Take advantage of the new "*trans*-free" spreads. Some even come enriched with the heart-healthy goodness of omega-3s from flax seed oil (for more information, see Flax Seed on page 142).

# Milk

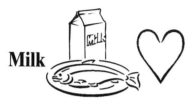

No doubt you've heard that "milk does a body good." But does milk do a heart good? Whether whole, reduced-fat (2%), low-fat (1%), or fat-free, milk is a stellar calcium source. A one-cup serving supplies about 30 percent of your need for this mineral which helps fight high-blood pressure. For years, scientists have noted that people with a poor intake of calcium seem to be at greater risk for developing hypertension. And likewise, people who regularly consume an adequate intake of calcium tend to have normal blood pressure. Milk may also have other protecting factors. Research shows that compared to non-milk drinkers, regular milk drinkers have a lower risk for serious strokes, often a result of chronic hypertension and heart disease.

In a landmark research project called the Honolulu Heart Program, researchers tracked a group of over 8000 men for the development of heart disease and stroke. The researchers were interested in what factors put some men at risk for heart disease and stroke and what factors were protective. Study participants were interviewed about their eating habits, specifically how much milk, if any, they drank daily.

Researchers found that risk for stroke was two times greater in men who didn't drink milk compared to men who consumed 16 ounces or more daily. It may be that milk drinking is associated with other healthful habits, but the researchers suspect that the milk's calcium and other nutrients provide protection against stroke.

However, you know as well as I do, that whole milk is loaded with fat. A one-cup serving contains about eight grams with a hefty five grams of it as cholesterol-raising saturated fat—25 percent of your Daily Value. And for those of you with risky blood cholesterol levels, your heart will thank you for switching to low-fat or fat-free milk. In fact, research shows that making the switch from whole milk to fat-free helps lower blood cholesterol levels. Scientists from the Department of Nutritional Sciences at the University of Washington put volunteers on a diet that contained about two and a half cups of either whole milk or fat-free milk. Within a month and a half of drinking fat-free milk, blood cholesterol levels fell significantly compared to those drinking whole milk.

Beyond the calcium in milk that keeps your heart healthy, milk is also a fabulous source of vitamin $B_{12}$, supplying over 40 percent of your needs in a one-cup serving. Vitamin $B_{12}$ is involved, along with folate and vitamin $B_6$, in clearing an artery-damaging substance in the circulation called homocysteine. Milk's

## Moo Stats

| Milk (8 ounces) | Calories | Fat (gm) | Saturated Fat (gm) | Calcium (mg) |
|---|---|---|---|---|
| Whole milk | 150 | 8.2 | 5.1 | 291 |
| Reduced-fat milk (2%) | 121 | 4.7 | 2.9 | 297 |
| Low-fat milk (1%) | 102 | 2.6 | 1.6 | 300 |
| Fat-free milk (skim) | 86 | .4 | .3 | 302 |
| Buttermilk | 99 | 2.2 | 1.3 | 285 |
| Chocolate milk (1%) | 158 | 2.5 | 1.5 | 287 |
| Evaporated milk, whole | 338 | 19 | 11.6 | 658 |
| Evaporated milk, fat-free | 200 | .8 | 0 | 736 |
| Sweetened condensed milk | 984 | 264 | 16.8 | 864 |

*Source:* Manufacturers' Food Labels

substantial content of potassium, almost as much as one banana, may also help explain milk's ability to help lower high blood pressure.

Fat-free and 1% milk along with other dairy products like yogurt (see Yogurt on page 293) are a vital part of your Simple Six Eating Plan. I recommend you have at lease two servings of low-fat or fat-free milk or dairy products each day. If lactose intolerance keeps you from enjoying milk, reach for lactose-free dairy products or consult your physician about taking a digestive aid. Besides warding off heart disease and hypertension, milk as a regular part of your daily fare also fights off the debilitating bone disease osteoporosis.

Many of the people I work with on making their diets heart-healthy say forget it to fat-free milk. "I have to draw the line somewhere when it comes to taste!" one client complained. Some people feel fat-free milk tastes like water or has a bluish tinge they can't get past. If this sounds like you, then try one of the new fat-free milk brands that has Replace® added, an oat-flour fat replacement. Sold under various private brands, the oat-flour boosted skim milk looks and tastes like real whole milk. And to boot, you get some extra oat fiber to lower blood cholesterol levels.

Besides drinking an ice-cold glass of milk or pouring it over a bowl of your favorite cereal, use it to top a bowl of sliced strawberries, peaches, or other fresh fruit. I use fat-free milk as the liquid when cooking up hot cereal like oat bran or 9-grain. This gives your cereal a creamier texture. Use milk in cream soups (check out my recipe for "Cream" of Celery Soup on page 105) and in baked dishes such as scalloped potatoes. You can also add warmed milk to mashed potatoes for a smooth consistency. But perhaps my favorite way to get milk is in a milkshake! Try my chocolate milkshake recipe—it has a whopping 50 percent of your daily calcium needs with the simple addition of dry milk powder.

### *Chocolate Calcium-Blast Milkshake*

Put the following in this order into a blender:

3/4 cup light ice cream, vanilla

2 tbsp. chocolate syrup

3/4 cup fat-free milk

1/4 cup nonfat dry milk powder

5 ice cubes

Place a lid on top of the blender and blend for 1 minute making sure dry milk powder is evenly distributed and not stuck on walls of blender (if it is, turn off blender and use a spatula to scrape sides). Pour into two glasses immediately. Enjoy with a straw. Serves two.

| Nutrition Facts |
|---|
| Chocolate Calcium-Blast Milkshake |
| Serving Size 1 cup |

| Amount per Serving | |
|---|---|
| Calories 192         3 Calories from fat | |
| | % Daily Value |
| Total Fat 22g | 4% |
|    Saturated Fat 2g | 8% |
| Cholesterol 11mg | 4% |
| Sodium 182mg | 8% |
| Total Carbohydrate 34g | 11% |
|    Dietary Fiber 1g | 2% |
| Protein 10g | |
| Vitamin A 20%  •  Vitamin C 3% | |
| Calcium 36%  •  Iron 3% | |

# Miso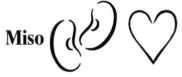

For centuries, the Japanese have used miso as an intense flavoring agent in clear broth soups and other traditional dishes. Miso is made from soybeans inoculated with a mold to initiate fermentation along with lots of sodium and a grain such as rice. This paste is then aged for a few years before it's ready for use.

But despite its sky-high sodium content (over 5000 milligrams in a half cup of miso!), miso has heart-disease fighting power from soybeans. The phytochemicals found in soy, called *isoflavones,* have been shown to lower blood cholesterol levels and heart-disease risk. And to boot, miso is packed with fiber, iron, and zinc along with folic acid to help lower the blood level of homocysteine which is known to damage artery walls and lead to heart disease.

The isoflavones found in miso help ward off heart disease in several ways. Studies show that these isoflavones, one in particular called *genistein,* help lower the "bad" carrier of cholesterol LDL. Also, genistein keeps LDLs from becoming oxidized, so they don't inflict damage on artery walls, leading to the development of heart disease. This means that as LDLs travel through your circulation, the chances are reduced that they end up driving like vehicles out of control into your blood vessel walls causing damage. Genistein also makes the blood vessel walls less sticky so that damaging particles are less likely to adhere and cause a blockage.

You can find miso at your local supermarket or Asian food store. Miso should be refrigerated after opening. Miso's intense flavor and high sodium content make it best suited as a seasoning agent or condiment. A tablespoon or two goes a long way for flavor. If you have salt-sensitive high blood pressure, you are better off using natto, a similar soybean paste that has virtually no sodium (see page 188).

Add miso to salad dressings or marinades for an intense flavor. Miso stirred into sauces and poured over grilled fish, chicken, or vegetables is also tasty. Or simply combine two tablespoons of miso into two cups of boiling water, stir, and add chopped scallions and enoki mushrooms (the thin, sprout-looking type) for warming, heart-healthy soup.

### Miso Marinade

*Goes best with salmon or swordfish.*

2 tbsp. of miso (light style)

1/4 cup sherry

1/4 cup honey

2 tbsp. pickled ginger (available in Asian food markets and some grocery stores)

2 tbsp. chopped garlic

Mix all the ingredients together in a bowl large enough to hold the fish. Use as a marinade; let fish sit 20 to 30 minutes and then grill or broil. Enough for one to two pounds of fish.

| **Nutrition Facts** | |
| --- | --- |
| Miso Marinade | |
| Serving Size 1/10 recipe | |
| **Amount per Serving** | |
| Calories 53      0 Calories from fat | |
| | % Daily Value |
| Total Fat 0g | 0% |
| Saturated Fat 0g | 0% |
| Cholesterol 0mg | 0% |
| Sodium 159mg | 7% |
| Total Carbohydrate 11g | 4% |
| Dietary Fiber <1g | 4% |
| Protein 1g | |
| Vitamin A 0% • Vitamin C 1% | |
| Calcium 1% • Iron 1% | |

# Molasses

The dark syrup leftover from extracting sugar crystals from sugar cane, molasses is sweet on your heart. Each two-tablespoon serving comes packed with a strong dose of the high blood pressure fighting mineral, calcium. Molasses also supplies 25 percent of your daily iron needs and all for only 95 calories and no fat. Not bad for an old-fashioned sweetener used since colonial times in traditional foods like Boston baked beans and gingerbread, and of course molasses cookies.

According to research, adding more calcium to your diet may help lower your blood pressure. In a study involving over 58,000 nurses, those routinely taking in more calcium in their diets had lower blood pressure than women who skimped on calcium intake. Another study from Japan showed that in over 1900 men, those eating more calcium had lower systolic blood pressure readings than men with low intakes of this mineral. Researchers suspect that calcium may, in part, counter the effects of a high sodium diet or may even relax the smooth muscles of the blood vessels making them more elastic.

You can use molasses as you would a sweetener but be prepared for a strong flavor and dark color. In place of brown sugar, top off cooked sweet potatoes or winter squash with a tablespoon or two of molasses. When making baked goods like dessert breads or cookies, replace some of the sugar with molasses. You can drizzle molasses over your hot cereal, yogurt, or even low-fat ice cream for a great taste. Try my molasses cookie recipe: I always have these on hand for a sweet, heart-healthy treat.

## *My Favorite Molasses Cookies*

2 cups unbleached flour

1/2 cup whole-wheat flour

1 tsp. baking soda

1 tsp. cinnamon

3/4 tsp. ginger

1/4 tsp. ground cloves

1/4 cup canola oil

1/4 cup soft *trans*-fat free margarine

1/2 cup brown sugar

1/4 cup reduced-fat egg substitute

1/2 cup molasses

1/2 cup buttermilk

In a medium-sized bowl, sift flours, baking soda, cinnamon, ginger, and cloves. Set aside. In a large bowl, beat together oil and margarine. Add brown sugar and continue beating. Add egg substitute and molasses and beat until light. Alternate flour mixture with buttermilk and mix into molasses mixture. Beat the batter until smooth. Drop by teaspoon onto a cookie sheet sprayed with a non-stick spray. Bake at 350 degrees for 8 to 11 minutes. Makes three dozen (two cookies per serving).

| Nutrition Facts | |
| --- | --- |
| Molasses Cookies | |
| Serving Size 2 cookies | |
| **Amount per Serving** | |
| Calories 159 | 54 Calories from fat |
| | % Daily Value |
| Total Fat 6g | 9% |
| Saturated Fat 1g | 4% |
| Cholesterol 0mg | 0% |
| Sodium 104mg | 4% |
| Total Carbohydrate 24g | 8% |
| Dietary Fiber 1g | 3% |
| Protein 3g | |
| Vitamin A 5% • Vitamin C 0% | |
| Calcium 8% • Iron 14% | |
| • Vitamin E 15% | |

# Mushrooms

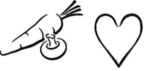

Not really a fruit or a vegetable, mushrooms are one of the most primitive life forms—fungi. And a tasty fungus it is. Chefs, gourmet cooks, and fans of fine food love mushrooms for their unique ability to enhance flavors. Mushrooms are a heart-healthy flavor booster thanks to their unusually high content of glutamic acid that acts in food very much like the well-known flavor enhancer MSG but without the sodium. And I love mushrooms for more than just their flavor. Mushrooms help lower high blood pressure as well as blood cholesterol levels.

Researchers from the Department of Food Chemistry at the University of Dhaka in Bangladesh put powdered shiitake and maitake mushrooms to the test. Special laboratory animals that are predisposed to hypertension, particularly when given excess salt in their diets, were fed dried mushrooms mixed in with their regular diet for about two months. Their blood pressure and cholesterol levels dropped significantly compared to animals who ate a mushroom-free diet. This and other research points to a magical, as yet undiscovered, substance in mushrooms that is responsible for its heart-healthy benefits.

Low in calories, about 20 per half cup cooked, and rich in potassium, mushrooms add great flavor to a variety of dishes. Fresh mushrooms, from the common white to the more exotic varieties such as enoki and portobello, are available year-round. Select fresh mushrooms that are free of serious pitting on the caps or spongy texture which indicates spoilage. You can also use dried mushrooms, which are quite flavorful when rehydrated in soups, stews, and casseroles.

Besides adding mushrooms to stir-fries and inside omelets, you can add raw mushrooms to salads, use the delicate enoki mushrooms as you would sprouts in sandwiches, or try adding at the last minute to broth soups. Larger mushrooms like portobello have a meaty texture that stands up well in stews or can even be grilled much like meat and served over risotto or polenta (cooked cornmeal). Try my recipe for portobello risotto. While these mushrooms are a bit pricey, their rich flavor and heart-healthy ingredients make them worth it!

### *Portobello Mushroom Risotto*

4 large portobello mushrooms, diced into cubes the size of thumb tip

3 cups of ariborio rice

8 cups of chicken stock

1 large onion, diced

4 cloves of garlic, chopped

4 tbsp. olive oil

Heat oil in a large cast iron skillet over medium heat. Add garlic and onion and cook until brown. Add portobello mushrooms and freshly ground pepper and sauté lightly for a few minutes. Mix in rice and cook another few minutes. Pour stock, 1 cup at a time every 4 minutes or so, over rice-mushroom mixture while stirring constantly. Continue stirring until rice is done. Serves ten.

| **Nutrition Facts** | |
|---|---|
| Portobello Mushroom Risotto | |
| Serving Size 1/10 recipe | |
| Amount per Serving | |
| Calories 301      63 Calories from fat | |
| | % Daily Value |
| Total Fat 7g | 11% |
| Saturated Fat 1g | 6% |
| Cholesterol 0mg | 0% |
| Sodium 625mg | 26% |
| Total Carbohydrate 49g | 16% |
| Dietary Fiber 2g | 6% |
| Protein 9g | |
| Vitamin A 0%   •   Vitamin C 5% | |
| Calcium 3%   •   Iron 19% | |

# Natto

Much like miso, natto is a soybean paste made from cooked soybeans with added grain, which is then (like cheese) inoculated with a bacteria for fermentation. Unlike miso, natto is virtually free of sodium and can be used more liberally in foods without worrying about high blood pressure. Natto's flavor is strong and somewhat cheese-like. Because natto is made from soybeans, it is packed with heart-disease fighting isoflavones.

A half-cup of natto (you may want to use less because of its strong flavor) has just over 180 calories and 9 grams of fat, with very little as saturated fat. Natto is also packed with fiber, about 20 percent of your daily needs, and an array of heart protecting nutrients. Each half cup also supplies a staggering 30 percent of magnesium, 25 percent of calcium, and 20 percent of potassium needs. That's a triple play for natto, as all of these minerals help ward off hypertension.

Natto is also a great source of protein, with 16 grams per serving (about 30 percent of your daily need). Since natto is made from soybeans, it has no cholesterol. Overall, you can't go wrong with adding some natto to your diet. It has a unique taste that I'll admit was unusual at first, but I quickly came to enjoy natto's sharp, tangy flavor.

Use natto as a topping over steamed rice or soban noodles, or toss into a vegetable stir-fry before serving. Natto can also be added to salads, especially cold grain salads such as cooked bulgur, brown rice, or barley. Add natto to soups, sauces, dressings, and marinades as you would use miso. Natto is sold in Asian food shops and in most ethnic food sections of supermarkets.

# Oats

Scientists got an inkling of oat's cholesterol-lowering powers back in the early 1960s. Since then, oats, specifically oatmeal and oat bran (the outer layer of whole oats) have been tops on the list of cholesterol busters. Thanks to a special fiber in oats called *beta-glucan,* cholesterol doesn't stand a chance. This water-soluble fiber acts like a piece of Velcro® in your intestinal tract by binding cholesterol and bile (made from cholesterol) and then making an exit with it in your stool. And the great news: You don't have to go on an oat-bran diet to get the benefits. Studies show that in some cases, as little as one bowl of oat bran cereal daily does the trick.

Cholesterol expert James Anderson, M.D., has put oat bran to the test in numerous studies using participants with high as well as normal blood cholesterol levels. In one study, subjects were fed a mere ounce of oat bran in the form of a ready-to-eat breakfast cereal for several weeks. This simple, yet effective change in diet pushed harmful levels of LDL down 8 percent. This may not seem like a sizable drop in LDL, but research shows it can have a significant impact on reducing heart disease.

Other studies consistently show that just two to three ounces of dry oat bran daily, equal to 1 1/2 to 2 1/2 cups of cooked oat bran cereal, lowers total cholesterol levels a staggering 15 to 20 percent and LDL levels from 12 to 24 percent in individuals with risky levels. And the beauty of oat fiber is that harmful cholesterol levels fall without lowering levels of the good-cholesterol carrier HDL.

Even people with healthy levels of cholesterol, below the 200 mark, may benefit from the beta-glucan in oats. In one study, LDL levels fell a whopping 23 percent in healthy subjects that added oat fiber to their daily diet. And you don't have to eat oat bran as cooked cereal to get its benefits. Research shows that oat bran lowers cholesterol levels whether eaten as cooked cereal, or as bread, muffins, or even as oat bran tablets.

Oats' powers in lowering your blood cholesterol level depends on where you start. Generally, the higher your initial starting point, that is, the riskier your reading, the greater it falls with the addition of oat fiber. Adding anywhere from one to three ounces of dry oat bran daily as cooked cereal or in other foods should push your cholesterol levels down. And along with other soluble fibers from beans and fruit as part of your Simple Six Eating Plan, your blood cholesterol levels will plummet.

### Oat Eats

Is cooked oatmeal and oat bran cereal the extent of your oat-eating cuisine? Like breakfast, that's just the beginning. You can get the goodness of oat fiber in just about every type of food imaginable. Use uncooked oatmeal as an ingredient in casseroles and stuffing mixes for poultry, fish, and vegetables such as bell

# Oat 'Riffic Cereal

These cereals work wonders on blood cholesterol.
Also included are cookies, muffins, and snacks.

| *Oat Products* | *Serving Size* | *Calories* | *Total Fiber (gm)* | *Soluble Fiber (gm)* | *Fat (gm)* |
|---|---|---|---|---|---|
| *Cereals* | | | | | |
| Quaker Oat Bran | 1 1/4 cup | 210 | 6 | 3 | 3 |
| Kellogg's Cracklin' Oat Bran | 3/4 cup | 190 | 6 | 0 | 6 |
| General Mills Cheerios | 1 cup | 110 | 3 | 1 | 2 |
| Kashi | 1/2 cup | 170 | 6 | na | 3 |
| *Hot Cereals* | | | | | |
| Quaker Instant Oatmeal | 1 packet | 100 | 3 | 1 | 2 |
| Sun Country Quick Oats | 1/2 cup | 150 | 4 | 2 | 3 |
| *Oat Cookies* | | | | | |
| Health Valley (33 gm) | 3 cookies | 100 | 3 | na | 0 |
| Mother's Old Fashioned Oatmeal Cookies | 2 cookies (26 gm) | 110 | 1 | na | 4.5 |
| *Oat Muffins* | | | | | |
| Krustaez Oat Bran (44 gm) | 1 muffin | 190 | 2 | na | 5 |
| Krustaez Low-Fat Apple Oat Bran | 1 muffin (50 gm) | 170 | 4 | 2 | 2 |
| *Snack Foods* | | | | | |
| Nutri-Grain (37 gm) | 1 bar | 140 | 1 | na | 3 |
| Nature Valley Crunch Granola Bars, cinnamon | 2 bars (42 gm) | 180 | 2 | na | 6 |

*Source:* Manufacturers' Food Labels (na = not available)

peppers. Oat bran can also be used as a coating for oven-baked chicken, fish, or eggplant. Simply dip chicken piece into buttermilk or egg substitute, then role into oat bran and bake as directed. It will be crunchy on the outside, deliciously juicy on the inside.

Baked goods including bread, cookies, and muffins make a smooth transition to heart-healthy treats with the addition of oat bran. (Check out "Feelin' Your Oats" on this page for a description of the types of oats available.) I like using uncooked oat bran and whole rolled oats as a crumb topping for baked apple crisp. The cholesterol-busting power of oats' beta-glucan along with apple's heart-saving flavonoids make this a steady dessert in our house. Try it topped with vanilla low-fat ice cream and there will never be enough.

Take advantage of the many recipes and cooking tips available from the oat-gurus themselves, Quaker Oats. Rolled oats and oat bran are sold in the cereal section of your local supermarket. On the backside of these packages are recipes along with information on how to send for more.

## Feelin' Your Oats

Here's the rundown on the different types of oats you can purchase for cooking and baking.

- *Steel-cut:* Often sold in bulk at health food stores, steel-cut oats (sometimes called Irish or Scotch oats) are the oat grain with the outer hulls removed and then cut into coarse pieces. Steel cut oats take longer to cook than regular oats, about 20 minutes, but they have a nice chewy texture.

- *Rolled:* These are dehulled oats that have been cooked slightly with steam and then are pressed flat with rollers. Cooking time is much less than steel-cut oats, about 5 minutes.

- *Instant:* These are precooked oats that have been pressed thin. Add boiling water and, ta-da, you have oatmeal.

## Oaty Apple Crisp

8 large Pippin or Granny Smith cooking apples, cored and sliced to 1/4-inch

1 1/2 cups rolled oats

3/4 cup brown sugar

3/4 cup chopped walnuts

1 tsp. sugar

2 tbsp. butter

3 tbsp. low-fat milk

Arrange apple slices in a 13- x 9-inch baking dish. Depending on the size of the apples you may need more (or less) to fill the dish just shy of the rim. In a separate bowl, mix all the dry ingredients with a fork using slicing-like motions. Cut butter into the mixture. Finally, drizzle milk over the top and mix. The mixture should be crumbly. Cover the top of the apple slices with this topping, making sure to pat down. Cover with foil and place in a 350-degree oven for 45 minutes. Remove foil and bake until apples appear bubbly at the bottom of the dish. Serves eight to ten. (I like to top a warm piece with nonfat ice cream.)

| **Nutrition Facts** | |
|---|---|
| Oaty Apple Crisp | |
| Serving Size 1/10 recipe | |
| **Amount per Serving** | |
| Calories 290  81 Calories from fat | |
| | % Daily Value |
| Total Fat 9g | 14% |
| Saturated Fat 2g | 11% |
| Cholesterol 6mg | 2% |
| Sodium 9mg | 0% |
| Total Carbohydrate 52g | 17% |
| Dietary Fiber 6g | 22% |
| Protein 4g | |
| Vitamin A 4%  •  Vitamin C 17% | |
| Calcium 5%  •  Iron 9% | |

# Olive Oil

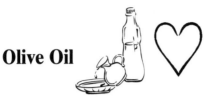

Rich in history, and even richer in heart-healthy benefits, olive oil is the "king" of oils and plays a vital part in your Simple Six Eating Plan. For thousands of years, olive oil has been part of our culinary heritage. A traditional Mediterranean diet, eaten for hundreds of years in countries such as Italy and Greece, revolves around olive oil. Tossed in fresh greens, over warm pasta, and as a "dip" for bread, olive oil makes up a substantial portion of total calories from fat, about a third of the daily calories. But despite a hefty fat intake, rates of heart disease are two to three times lower in these countries than in the U.S. where fat intake is lower.

The secret lies in the type of fat. Olive oil is rich (over 70 percent) in monounsaturated fats. This type of fat (also found, but in lower amounts, in avocado, canola, and peanut oils) lowers blood cholesterol levels, appears to protect the LDL cholesterol carriers from oxidizing and damaging artery walls, while also lowering blood pressure and reducing the risk of heart disease. Need I say more? Olive oil is a must in your diet.

### The Evidence

A staggering number of research studies from around the world suggest that olive oil works wonders on your heart. In a landmark study carried out in the 1950s and 1960s, Mediterranean countries were found to have one-third to one-half the risk of dying from heart disease compared to the United States or other Northern European countries. When the researchers factored out cigarette smoking, high blood pressure, and other factors that can change heart-disease risk, they found that most of the difference in death rates could be explained by the use of olive oil and the lower saturated fat intake in the Mediterranean diets. In other words, for heart health cut back on saturated fats and use olive oil.

The secret to olive oil's heart-saving powers is its action on circulating cholesterol. Recall that cholesterol moves around your body as a passenger in different types of lipoprotein "buses." The LDL bus is the bad guy because elevated levels (too many buses) as well as oxidized or damaged LDLs lead to clogged arteries and heart disease. The HDL, on the other hand, is the good bus cleaning up loose cholesterol and taking it back to headquarters (the liver) for eventual excretion from the body. When olive oil takes the place of saturated fats in the diet, cholesterol levels drop in a most enchanted way. LDL levels go down (good news) and HDL levels either stay the same or go up (even better news).

In a study by Dr. Valentina Ruiz-Gutiérrez in Sevila, Spain, women with hypertension were put on an olive-oil rich diet for four weeks. Compared to a control period, total cholesterol levels dropped but the HDL cholesterol rose. To boot, the women's blood pressure dropped significantly while on the olive-oil enriched diet.

In other research, an olive-oil rich diet not only lowered the LDL level but also provided some protection to the LDLs against oxidation, making LDLs less likely to stick to artery walls. Researchers guess that once the fat in olive oil becomes part of the LDL structure, the LDL becomes more stable, less harmful, and not as likely to break down and become oxidized.

### Well Oiled

All this good news about olive oil may prompt you to douse everything in this wondrous elixir. But before you rush out and buy a jug, keep in mind that olive oil has calories, and lots of them: 114 per tablespoon serving. And despite olive oil's heart-healthy reputation, too much of a good thing can lead to unwanted weight gain. As Carl found out, pouring olive oil on cooked pasta, potatoes, and vegetables along with dipping bread, crackers, and bagels in the stuff, while well intentioned, boosts calorie intake. He put on a few pounds over a month's time, and we both pinpointed his olive-oil slathering as the culprit. So be sure to keep amounts within the Simple Six Eating Plan framework for your calorie intake (see Chapter Two, page 22, for more details).

When selecting olive oil, consider its use and a price range your wallet can handle. Olive oil comes in several varieties— "Extra Virgin," "Virgin," "Light," and others. Find a description of each in the "Oil Change" chart. The major way these varieties differ is in the amount of acidity in each. During the pressing of olives, some breakdown in the fat, called a *triglyceride,* occurs. As a result, some of the attached fatty acid is set free, giving the oil a measurable acidity. Thus the lower the acidity level, the better the quality because less damage has occurred.

Olive oil types vary in flavor as well, not only from the type of olive (where it is grown, etc.), but also from the amount of olive particles in the oil (usually from second and third pressings) which impart a distinct flavor that you may or may not want. Olive oil that is well filtered can be used like conventional oils (corn or safflower oils) in baking without imparting an "olivey" taste.

Use olive oil as you would any other added fat. But know that a little goes a long way when it comes to flavor. Using olive oil in a vegetable sauté, for example, gives a Truscan-like flair without using much oil. And this is where price comes into play. Olive oil typically costs more than most vegetable oils, but a little goes a long way. Save more exquisite brands of olive oil for a special meal where flavor is of the utmost; and keep a generic, less-costly variety on hand for everyday use, such as bread dipping and salad dressings.

Olive oil is a fabulous addition drizzled over fresh green salads, roasted vegetables or potatoes, pasta with or without sauce, in marinades for tofu, chicken, and beef, and as an ingredient in dressing for salads, sauces, and more. (Try my vinaigrette recipe.) But drizzling olive oil out of a bottle is a fine art. If you're like me, olive oil glugs out of the bottle rather than drizzles and I get more than I asked for. Try an oil sprayer if drizzling is not an art form you have mastered. Sprayers are available at gourmet cook shops; simply pour in your favorite brand of oil and spray. It gives you a light mist that evenly coats foods, pans, skillets, anything you want. This kitchen gadget is worth the $20 price tag. See my recipe for Oven Potato "Fries" using an oil mister.

## *Vinaigrette for Fresh Greens*

5 tbsp. olive oil

5 tbsp. red wine vinegar

1 clove crushed garlic or very finely chopped

freshly ground pepper to taste

salt or salt substitute to taste

Combine all ingredients in a jar with a tightly fitting lid and shake vigorously before using. Use one to two tablespoons per serving. Start with less, you can always add more. Refrigerate unused portion.

**Variations:** You can add a wide array of ingredients to "customize" your vinaigrette: horseradish, tabasco sauce, curry powder, fresh herbs such as rosemary or dill, anchovy paste, and mustard, to name a few.

---

**Nutrition Facts**

Vinaigrette for Fresh Greens

Serving Size 1 tablespoon

| Amount per Serving | |
|---|---|
| Calories 61 | 61 Calories from fat |
| | % Daily Value |
| Total Fat 7g | 10% |
| Saturated Fat 1g | 5% |
| Cholesterol 0mg | 0% |
| Sodium 0mg | 0% |
| Total Carbohydrate 0g | 0% |
| Dietary Fiber 0g | 0% |
| Protein 0g | |

| | | |
|---|---|---|
| Vitamin A 0% | • | Vitamin C 0% |
| Calcium 0% | • | Iron 0% |

## Oven Potato "Fries"

4 large baking potatoes (Russet)

olive oil in oil spray bottle (Misto® brand)

salt to taste (optional)

Wash potatoes, removing any bad spots. Poke a few holes in each with a sharp knife and microwave on high power for 5 minutes. Remove and cut each potato in half lengthwise and then cut each half into lengthwise wedges about a half-inch wide. Arrange on baking sheet and spray with oil (total amount of oil used about 2 tablespoons) and salt if desired. Bake at 400 degrees until potatoes are golden brown and soft, about 15 to 20 minutes.

**Variations:** Sprinkle with Parmesan cheese during the last five minutes of baking, or sprinkle with garlic powder or herb seasoning halfway through baking. Makes eight servings.

## Nutrition Facts

Oven Potato "Fries"

Serving Size 1/2 potato prepared

| Amount per Serving | |
|---|---|
| Calories 140      27 Calories from fat | |
| | % Daily Value |
| Total Fat 3g | 5% |
| Saturated Fat 1g | 2% |
| Cholesterol 0mg | 0% |
| Sodium 8mg | 0% |
| Total Carbohydrate 26g | 9% |
| Dietary Fiber 2g | 9% |
| Protein 2g | |

| | |
|---|---|
| Vitamin A 0% | • Vitamin C 22% |
| Calcium 1% | • Iron 8% |
| | • Vitamin B$_6$ 18% |

## Oil Change

Confused about the different "grades" of olive oil? Here's a rundown on their differences and uses.

- *Extra Virgin:* Oil from the first pressing of olives, it is unrefined (not filtered) so usually has good "olive" green color. Only allowed 1% or less acid content, a measure of fat breakdown. Good for uses where a strong but delicate olive oil taste is wanted. Use in sautés, dressings, marinades.

- *Virgin:* Also from the first pressing and unrefined, but with a 4% acidity level; to the discerning palate a slightly harsher flavor. Use as with virgin olive oil.

- *Pure:* A mix of the first and second pressing, usually refined to remove substances that impart a harsh flavor. Not as flavorful as virgin or extra virgin but use the same way.

- *Light:* Not lower in fat or calories but "light" on olive oil flavor. The olive residue is removed so this oil can be used in baking as a substitute for other vegetable oil where an olive taste is not desired.

# Onions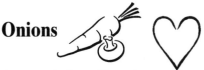

As a cousin to garlic, onions are true to their family (of vegetables, that is) and fight hard for your heart's health. When taking a quick look at onion's nutritional profile, you don't notice anything too outstanding—a bit of fiber, vitamin C, folate, potassium, and about 30 calories per half-cup raw. Take a longer look, though, and you find a host of powerful phytochemicals. These warriors against heart disease are called *flavonoids,* and according to several large research studies from around the world, they significantly reduce the risk of death from heart disease.

The standout flavonoid in onions, *quercitin,* has been shown experimentally to protect the bad cholesterol carriers, LDLs, from oxidizing and damaging artery walls. In addition, quercitin also keeps blood from getting too sticky and jamming up blood vessels leading to an actual heart attack or stroke. In a Finish study, women with the greatest intake of quercitin from onions had half the risk of dying from heart disease compared to women in the study with the lowest intake. The researchers suspect the quercitin performed its two-pronged magic to protect the women from a fatal heart attack.

Quercitin levels in onions depend on their color. White onions have next to nothing in the way of this phytochemical, while yellow and red or Bermuda onions are packed with quercitin. Since onions are so versatile, they can be added to almost every dish—raw or cooked.

If the strong odor of onions bothers you, thanks to similar sulfur compounds responsible for garlic's aroma, try some of the sweeter onion varieties that have less of these offensive chemicals. Red onions usually from California, Walla Wallas from Washington, and Vidalias from Georgia are sweeter than standard yellow onions and can be used raw in salads and on sandwiches. The Maui onion from Hawaii is so sweet, you can eat it like you would a piece of fruit off a tree.

Select onions that are hard and firm without soft spots, and that are not beginning to sprout. Always store onions in a dark, cool, dry place such as a basement, cool pantry, or cellar. Putting an onion in the refrigerator about 30 minutes before slicing or chopping will help reduce the amount of tearing you may endure when preparing onions. When an onion is broken open, an enzyme-driven process causes a chemical to form. This irritant is volatile and travels in the air to your eyes, making you weepy. You can avoid wet eyes by doing your onion chopping in a food processor.

Use onions in soups, stews, casseroles, pasta dishes, and side dishes such as cooked rice, potatoes, and corn. Chopped onions work well as a topping for pizza and baked potato, or inside an omelet or stuffed bell pepper. Toss raw onions into green salads, salsas (fruit salsas included), or top off a sandwich, veggie burger, or grilled fish with raw onion slices. Try my onion-topped pizza for a good dose of quercitin for your heart.

## *Onion-Topped Pizza*

2 large onions sliced in thin rings

2 cloves of garlic, chopped

2 tsp. fresh rosemary

2 tbsp. olive oil

1 large pizza shell, thin crust (unbaked)

1 oz. grated Parmesan cheese

2 tomatoes, sliced

In a skillet, heat oil over medium heat and add onions, garlic, and rosemary. Sauté until caramelized. Remove from heat and spread onion mixture over pizza shell. Sprinkle cheese on top. Place pizza on a cookie sheet and bake in a 400-degree oven for 15 to 20 minutes, until crust is done. Top with tomato slices and serve. Makes eight servings.

| **Nutrition Facts** | |
|---|---|
| Onion-Topped Pizza | |
| Serving Size 1/8 recipe | |
| **Amount per Serving** | |
| Calories 215      58 Calories from fat | |
| | % Daily Value |
| Total Fat 6g | 10% |
| Saturated Fat 1g | 6% |
| Cholesterol 3mg | 1% |
| Sodium 70mg | 3% |
| Total Carbohydrate 32g | 11% |
| Dietary Fiber 2g | 8% |
| Protein 7g | |
| Vitamin A 3%    •    Vitamin C 13% | |
| Calcium 10%    •    Iron 29% | |

# Oranges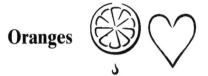

Perhaps one of Mother Nature's best super foods, an orange comes packed with an unbelievable array of heart disease and high blood pressure fighting nutrients, all tucked neatly underneath a bright orange peel. A medium orange has a mere 70 calories loaded with 130 percent of your vitamin C needs, over 20 percent of fiber, and 12 percent of folate along with a good dose of potassium. All these nutrients along with a hefty arsenal of phytochemicals make oranges a must for your Simple Six Eating Plan.

The vitamin C in oranges has been shown to be effective in both lowering blood cholesterol levels and protecting the cholesterol-carrying LDLs from becoming damaging to artery walls. Researchers in Israel supplied a group of men with enough freshly squeezed orange juice daily to provide 500 milligrams of vita-min C (about 40 ounces). Following two months of this or-ange-supplemented diet, researchers noted that the men's LDLs stayed intact and did not become oxidized or "hostile," meaning they were safer to artery walls compared to a group of men who did not drink the orange juice daily.

An array of studies have shown that the fiber in oranges, called *pectin,* is very effective in lowering blood cholesterol levels. Pectin's benefits are even more dramatic in people with blood cholesterol levels in the danger zone. The folate in oranges, according to research, plays an important role in clearing away homocysteine from the circulation. Even though this protein-like substance is produced by our bodies normally, homocysteine is considered dangerous for blood vessels if levels get too high. In fact, people who skimp on folate in their diet have greater levels of circulating homocysteine and potentially a greater risk for heart disease.

Oranges also contain flavonoids, a type of phytochemical that protects your heart. Flavonoids have been shown to protect LDLs from oxidizing and to keep blood cells from becoming sticky and glopping up in blood vessels causing a heart attack. Also, one phytochemical in particular, *limone*—only found in oranges and other citrus—is a particularly powerful antioxidant that protects your heart. This helps explain why people who regularly eat a diet rich in oranges and other citrus fruits have a lower risk for heart disease.

Much of the orange's fiber and phytochemicals, particularly the flavonoids, are found both in the pulpy part of the orange and in the white fuzzy stuff just under the orange peel, called the *albedo layer.* Eating a freshly peeled orange without painstakingly pulling off the albedo layer is the best way to get all of the heart-healthy powers of an orange. Orange juice often has much of the pulp and albedo filtered out and is typically much lower in fiber than a whole orange and lower in phytochemicals too.

Great news about oranges: They are available year-round in your grocery store's produce section. Select fruit that is firm and heavy for its size which indicates good juice content. Avoid spongy or mushy feeling oranges, a sign of spoilage or very thick skins without much inside. Oranges go well with all types of dishes—appetizers, salads, main dishes (especially chicken), and of course, desserts. My Orange 'n Bean Salad makes a colorful side dish for barbecued chicken, fish or tofu. Oranges are staples around my house; I eat at least two every day! My family's favorite is our one-minute orange-vanilla morning smoothie. Throw peeled oranges and low-fat frozen yogurt or soy milk in a blender with ice cubes and a splash of vanilla. Or you can always enjoy a freshly peeled orange and that soothing orange aroma that comes with it—one of life's simple pleasures.

### Orange 'n Bean Salad

2 oranges, peeled and cut into slices (circle) and then in half

1 can garbanzo beans, drained

1 can kidney beans, drained

1 small or 1/2 large red onion, cut into slices, then in half and separated into strips

zest of half an orange (use one of the oranges before peeling)

1/4 cup reduced-fat Italian salad dressing

1 tbsp. olive oil

1 tbsp. balsamic vinegar

1/4 tsp. ground pepper

In a bowl combine oranges, beans, and onions. In a small jar with lid, combine the remaining ingredients and shake vigorously to blend. Pour over orange mixture and toss until evenly distributed. Serve with fresh coriander garnish. Serves six.

| **Nutrition Facts** | |
| :--- | ---: |
| Orange 'n Bean Salad | |
| Serving Size 1/6 recipe | |
| **Amount per Serving** | |
| Calories 119      36 Calories from fat | |
| | % Daily Value |
| Total Fat 4g | 6% |
| Saturated Fat <1g | 2% |
| Cholesterol 0mg | 0% |
| Sodium 301mg | 13% |
| Total Carbohydrate 20g | 7% |
| Dietary Fiber 4g | 16% |
| Protein 5g | |
| Vitamin A 1%   •   Vitamin C 48% | |
| Calcium 4%   •   Iron 6% | |
| •   Vitamin E 17% | |

# Oysters

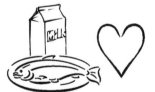

Along with pearls, oysters give us a gift of even greater value—a healthy heart. These shellfish come loaded (and I mean loaded!) with key nutrients for your heart. A modest serving of six medium-sized oysters, about one and a half ounces, supplies a staggering

700 percent of your vitamin $B_{12}$ needs and 500 percent of the mineral zinc. Besides this, oysters contain heart-healthy omega-3 fats shown to fight heart disease and lower high blood pressure.

Vitamin $B_{12}$, along with the vitamins folate and $B_6$, are involved in clearing the artery-damaging blood factor called homocysteine. And since your body's ability to use $B_{12}$ tends to decline with age, you can always use a $B_{12}$ boost. That's where a bowl of steamed oysters makes good sense for your heart. The zinc in oysters also helps protect your heart. This mineral works with a special enzyme inside cells called SOD (short for *superoxide dismutase*) responsible for protecting your cells from damage caused by free radicals. And it is this type of oxidative damage that causes destruction to artery walls leading to heart disease.

There's more! Oysters' heart-healing powers continue with their offering of omega-3 fats. Each serving has just under a gram of these fish oils that research shows not only help lower blood fat levels, but may even reduce the risk of sudden cardiac arrest. A study published in the *Journal of the American Medical Association* demonstrated that eating what amounts to three ounces of oysters per week reduced the risk of sudden cardiac arrest caused by the twitching, referred to as fibrillation, of the heart muscle.

And as an aside, don't worry about the cholesterol level in oysters, about 40 milligrams in a serving. Two-thirds of this is a type of sterol (cholesterol relative) that actually blocks cholesterol absorption into the body. All things considered, oysters' great heart-healthy profile makes them a fabulous addition to your Simple Six Eating Plan.

When buying fresh oysters, make sure to shop at a busy, reputable fish market or grocery store. Since oysters take in gallons of sea water everyday as a way of eating, there is a chance that harmful bacteria or other pathogens may be picked up. This is a good reason to stay away from raw oysters. Oysters should be harvested from state-certified waters which is at least some reassurance of reduced contamination risk. Always eat oysters cooked; steam until their edges curl but don't overcook as this makes them tough. If you're in a hurry, you can eat cooked oysters right out of the can (balance on your favorite cracker or simply pluck one with a toothpick). Oysters make great additions to soups, seafood stews, and pasta dishes.

# Papaya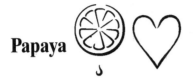

A slice of paradise, papaya has a peachy-melon like flavor that comes packed with a trio of heart-saving nutrients. Just half of a medium-sized papaya supplies a whopping 150 percent of your vitamin C needs and a good dose of the B vitamin, folate, along with cryptoxanthin, a type of carotene that gives papaya flesh its orange-rose color. That's not bad for only 60 calories!

Cryptoxanthin (pronounced *crip-toe-zan-theen*) works wonders protecting your heart from oxidative damage. Researchers believe that this and other carotenes actually help reduce destruction to artery walls. In one study, laboratory animals that are particularly prone to developing heart disease were fed diets supplemented with papayas and guavas, another tropical fruit rich in carotenes. Following six months of treatment, animals developed fewer fatty deposits and damaged arteries with the papaya-guava diet than without.

The vitamin C in papaya also protects your heart and helps keep blood pressure levels in check. Studies show that people who routinely get more vitamin C in their diets have greater levels of the cholesterol-scavenging HDLs which help flush cholesterol from the body by way of the liver. Also, higher circulating levels of vitamin C are linked with lower blood pressure. This good news makes papayas a natural for your fruit bowl at home.

Papayas, shaped much like a large pear, are typically available year-round in the produce section. Depending on the amount of green showing, papayas ripen in about two to seven days when left in a fruit bowl at room temperature. You can speed this up by placing a papaya in a paper bag. A ripe papaya is slightly soft to the touch and has a golden-yellow appearance with a touch of green. Cut one open and you'll find yellow-gold to rose-orange flesh with a center of small black seeds. Once peeled you can toss sliced papaya into salsas, fruit salads, green salads, as well as cold seafood or pasta salads. My tropical smoothie recipe gives you the heart-warming goodness of soy and papaya. Or simply enjoy the summer sweet bouquet of a ripe papaya all by itself. Peel, slice, and drizzle with lemon juice for a treat you will want to repeat.

## *Island Blast*

1/2 ripe papaya, seeds removed

1/2 ripe banana

juice from 1 lime

1/2 cup lemonade

1 tbsp. shredded coconut

5 ice cubes

1 oz. isolated soy protein powder, nonflavored (use two ounces if flavored version is used)

2 tsp. honey

Put all the ingredients in a blender, put lid on, and blend on high until well mixed. Taste before serving as it may need more sweetener—honey or your choice of artificial sweetener such as Equal®. Makes two servings (one serving counts as one soy serving).

## Nutrition Facts

Island Blast

Serving Size 1/2 recipe

| Amount per Serving | |
|---|---|
| Calories 166    10 Calories from fat | |
| | % Daily Value |
| Total Fat 1g | 2% |
| Saturated Fat 1g | 5% |
| Cholesterol 0mg | 0% |
| Sodium 154mg | 6% |
| Total Carbohydrate 28g | 9% |
| Dietary Fiber 2g | 9% |
| Protein 13g | |

Vitamin A 15% • Vitamin C 100%
Calcium 15% • Iron 14%
• Vitamin E 84%

# Pasta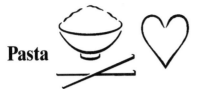

With names like spaghetti and linguine, you can't help but think pasta had its origins in Italy. China, however, is actually where this unleavened (no yeast), flour-water dough was first made into dumpling-like noodles. But Italy popularized pasta as a dietary staple. By the 18th century, Italians figured out mass production of pasta, eventually eliminating the need for individual households to make fresh pasta daily. And today, we have literally hundreds of different shapes and colors of pasta that entertain sauces and toppings of all kinds. It's wonderful that such a versatile, economic, and convenient food is also good for your heart.

A half-cup serving of cooked pasta, equal to one ounce dry before cooking, supplies a good dose of complex carbohydrates along with B vitamins including folate, all in only 100 calories. Pasta that is made with whole-wheat flour also supplies fiber, about three grams per serving or 12 percent of your daily need. Some pastas have vegetable purées or powders (spinach, beets, carrots) added, which perks up the pasta's color but not much in the way of extra nutrition because such a small amount is used. The term *pasta* embraces two categories: macaroni, which is a pasta made from a flour-water combination; and noodles, which are essentially macaroni with eggs (typically powdered) added to the mix before pasta shapes are formed.

It's pasta's carbohydrate content that most likely gives it a heart-healthy glow. Studies show that in countries such as Italy, where intake of carbohydrate from pasta and other grain products is high, the risk of heart disease is low. Scientists that track types of foods and related health benefits theorize that a high carbohydrate diet as opposed to one high in fat, lowers heart-disease risk by keeping fat off the dinner plate.

In one study from Harvard School of Medicine, subjects' blood cholesterol levels fell while eating a diet supplemented with low-fiber complex carbohydrate foods such as plain or white pasta or rice. The cholesterol plunge in these subjects most likely occurred because they ate less fat while beefing up their carbohy-drate intake. And lowering fat in your diet can have a big impact on lowering blood cholesterol levels and lessening the risk for heart disease.

View pasta as one of those gotta-have-on-hand foods. Your cupboards or pantry should have at least two different types of dry pasta. Fresh pasta sold in the refrigerator section of most grocery stores is as nutritious as dry pasta. Stored in the refrigerator, fresh pasta keeps a few weeks (check date on package) or you can freeze it for up to six months. Fresh pasta cooks up in minutes (usually less than five to seven minutes) and dry pasta is ready in 10 to 18 minutes. So either version, wet or dry, is convenient.

One look at the "Pasta Shop" chart and you can appreciate the variety of pastas available. Try different shapes and see how

## Pasta Shop

The array of pasta shapes can be confusing. Here's a description of several to help in your selection.

- Angel's Hair or Capelline D'Angelo—very thin strands of pasta.
- Agnolotti—crescent moon-shaped filled pasta.
- Farfalle—bow tie- or butterfly-shaped pasta.
- Fettuccine—flat strands of pasta.
- Fusilli—pasta shaped in spirals.
- Linguine—a narrower version of fettuccine.
- Penne—tube-shaped pasta with diagonally cut ends.
- Ravioli—square or rectangular stuffed pasta.
- Rigatoni—a larger version of penne.
- Rotelle—spiral-shaped pasta (or wagon wheel).
- Rotini—spiral-shaped pasta.
- Spaghetti—round strands of pasta (a basic shape that works with most sauces).
- Tortellini—small, crescent-shaped filled pasta.
- Ziti—tube-shaped pasta.

you like them for their sauce "holding" capacity. When selecting whole-grain pasta, keep in mind that it has a chewy texture, so at first, start with smaller shapes until your eating audience is accustomed to the flavor and texture.

Filled pastas, such as ravioli and tortellini, come with their insides stuffed with cheese, vegetables like spinach, and meats including chicken and even crab. These fillings can add protein, and other nutrients, but often add extra fat. Check the label on these fresh and frozen varieties for fat and saturated fat grams per serving. You're better off, in some cases, topping plain pasta with your choice of ingredients.

Topping cooked pasta is your chance to have some fun and be artistic at the same time, as you create a glorious medley of tastes, textures, and temperatures. Dress pasta with fresh, low-fat ingredients. Lightly steamed vegetables—broccoli, asparagus, greens—along with a touch of fresh garlic and a splash of olive oil make a simple heart-healthy dish. Toss in cooked shrimp, salmon, tofu, or strips of chicken or beef. Leftover pasta is great reheated with a red sauce and a touch of Parmesan cheese. Cold pasta salads, fun-shaped pasta (I like the bow ties) mixed with sugar peas, carrots, cabbage, and sprigs of coriander, are a cool but heart-warming dinner at our house during the dog days of summer.

## Chili-Style Pasta

*I am almost embarrassed at how easy this dish is to make, but it's always a favorite.*

1 12-oz. package of penne pasta or other tube or spiral-shaped pasta (cooks to about 6 cups)

1 can vegetarian chili

1 can beef and bean chili (Denison brand), 99% fat-free

toppings: grated reduced-fat cheddar cheese, chopped tomatoes, chopped onions, nonfat sour cream

In a big pot, cook pasta as directed on package and drain and return to pot. In another saucepan, mix together both types of chili and heat through. Toss chili into pasta pot and stir. Serve in bowl and top with your choice of toppings. Serves six to eight.

---

**Nutrition Facts**

Chili-Style Pasta

Serving Size 1 1/4 cups

---

Amount per Serving

---

Calories 239      11 Calories from fat

---

| | % Daily Value |
|---|---|
| Total Fat 1g | 2% |
|    Saturated Fat <1g | 2% |
| Cholesterol 9mg | 3% |
| Sodium 619mg | 26% |
| Total Carbohydrate 44g | 15% |
|    Dietary Fiber 5g | 21% |
| Protein 12g | |

---

| Vitamin A 5% | • | Vitamin C 1% |
|---|---|---|
| Calcium 3% | • | Iron 11% |

---

# Peanuts

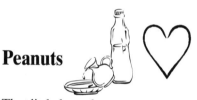

That little bag of peanuts you get on an airplane may actually be a heart saver. Peanuts are really not nuts at all but legumes like navy or kidney beans. Legumes protect your heart in much the same way as red wine may. The artery-guardian phytochemical called *resveratrol* found in red wine is also in peanuts. But peanuts' goodness goes beyond resveratrol.

Peanuts are high in fat, 14 grams per one-ounce serving, which is about a handful. But much of this fat is cholesterol-lowering monounsaturated fat. According to many research studies, diets rich in monounsaturated fats lower heart-disease risk. In fact, studies show that when peanut oil replaces saturated fats such as butter in the diet, cholesterol levels fall. Peanuts also supply about

20 percent of your vitamin E needs per serving, the vitamin responsible for protecting your arteries from damaging LDLs, along with a dose of folate, a B vitamin that helps protect your heart.

The news for regular peanut munching is good. In a study from Loma Linda University in California, more than 30,000 women were interviewed extensively about their dietary habits. Women who ate peanuts and other nuts four times a week or more had half the risk for fatal and nonfatal heart attacks compared to women eating peanuts less than once a week. Other research studies, such as one in Iowa with 40,000 women, also support frequent peanut-eating as a heart saving measure.

Peanuts are best eaten raw, that is, unroasted with no added salt, with their red skins, a good source of resveratrol. Because raw peanuts haven't been heat-treated, they are a better source of vitamin E than roasted varieties. If you haven't sampled raw peanuts, you're in for a taste treat. In their untreated state, peanuts have more of a pea-like flavor. When selecting roasted peanuts, reach for dry roasted rather than those roasted in oils (oftentimes hydrogenated vegetable oils). And skip the salted ones if you're watching your blood pressure.

My favorite, peanut butter, is a great way to get the heart-healthy goodness of peanuts. Like other nut butters (see "Going Nuts" chart), peanut butter is a great source of vitamin E. Select

## Going Nuts

Nut butters made from ground peanuts, almonds, hazelnuts, and others make for heart-healthy spreads on everything from plain bread to apple slices.

| Nut Butter (2 Tbsp.) | Vitamin E (mg) | % Daily Value |
|---|---|---|
| Peanut butter | 3.2 | 32 |
| Cashew butter | 0.5 | 5 |
| Almond butter | 6.5 | 65 |
| Hazelnut butter | 6.8 | 68 |

brands that use fresh, whole ground peanuts without added sugar, hydrogenated vegetable oils, or other additives. Most peanut butters come with added salt, so again, check levels if reducing sodium in the diet helps control your blood pressure. Many health food stores offer "make-your-own" peanut butter. Simply pour the desired amount of roasted peanuts into a grinder and press start. Freshly made peanut butter on a slice of whole-wheat bread is my idea of a hearty but heavenly snack!

You can add peanuts to cold salads, top your morning cereal, or as a tasty addition to casseroles. Many Thai recipes call for peanuts. They make a great complement to some of the fiery spices used in Thai cuisine. Try my Peanut Sauce recipe for grilled chicken skewers, from a good friend, Mumulay, a chef whose roots are in Indonesia.

### *Peanut Sauce*

*Great for dipping grilled seafood, spring rolls, and potstickers.*

1 clove of garlic, crushed

1-inch cube of fresh ginger (peeled)

1 small yellow onion, peeled and cut in quarters

1/2 cup vegetable broth

2 small tomatoes, chopped

3 tbsp. creamy peanut butter

1/3 cup soft tofu

juice from 1 lime

1 tbsp. reduced-sodium soy sauce

1/4 tsp. red pepper flakes (or use chili paste)

In a food processor, combine garlic, ginger, and onion and process until finely chopped. In a saucepan, add broth and garlic mixture. Bring to a boil and then reduce heat, allowing mixture to simmer until the liquid has evaporated down to about one-third. Combine peanut butter, lime juice, soy sauce, and pepper flakes in food processor and blend. Add, along with chopped tomatoes, to garlic-broth mixture. Simmer until sauce has thickened (about 10–15 minutes). Serves four generously.

## Nutrition Facts
Peanut Sauce
Serving Size 1/4 recipe

| Amount per Serving | |
|---|---|
| Calories 111     64 Calories from fat | |
| | % Daily Value |
| Total Fat 7g | 11% |
| Saturated Fat 1.3g | 7% |
| Cholesterol 0mg | 0% |
| Sodium 161mg | 7% |
| Total Carbohydrate 9g | 3% |
| Dietary Fiber 2g | 9% |
| Protein 6g | |

| | | |
|---|---|---|
| Vitamin A 5% | • | Vitamin C 24% |
| Calcium 3% | • | Iron 9% |
| | • | Vitamin E 21% |

 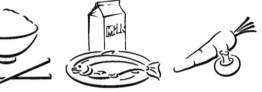

# Pizza

The phrase "health food" doesn't exactly come to mind when you think of pizza. Dripping with melted cheese, sausage, pepperoni, and other artery-clogging delights, an average two-slice serving of pizza packs over 400 calories and 25 grams of fat, half of which is cholesterol-raising saturated fat. But if you're a pizza fan (and who isn't), don't despair. From my perspective, pizza is a heart-healthy food; it's all in the way you slice it. Layered with the right toppings and loaded with the health benefits of tomato sauce, pizza slices up as a real heart-saver.

Whether ordering from a pizza joint, purchasing frozen pizza, or making your own, make sure not to skimp on the to-mato sauce. Tomatoes, especially in tomato sauce, are an excellent source of a carotene called *lycopene*. Studies show that lycopene works as a very powerful antioxidant protecting you from various age-related diseases such as cancer and heart disease. Once in your system, some lycopene gets tucked away in fat tissue, thus levels of lycopene in this tissue indicate intake of this carotene over time.

In one study, scientists from Germany sampled the lycopene content in fat tissue from men who suffered heart attacks and compared this to levels found in men who hadn't experienced a heart attack. The researchers found that the heart attack sufferers had lower levels of lycopene in fat tissue compared to the other men. In fact, men with the lowest levels of lycopene were about twice as likely to suffer from a heart attack as men with the greatest levels.

Besides the heart-healthy goodness of tomato sauce, pizza toppings can pack a nutritional punch as well. For starters, standard pizza cheese, mozzarella, is lower in fat than most cheeses such as cheddar and Monterey Jack. When ordering pizza, ask for less cheese to save on fat. When making your own, you can use low-fat or even nonfat cheeses (but be aware that the consistency of melted nonfat cheese is a bit different from the real thing).

What tops off the cheese makes your pizza either a heart saver or heart stopper. For vitamin, mineral, and fiber goodness, select vegetable toppings including sliced green and red peppers,

## Top It Off

Make pizza baking in your own home fast and heart healthy. Use pizza shells available in grocery stores (select those with less than five grams of fat per serving). Top with tomato sauce and reduced-fat mozzarella cheese. Then pile on goodies including:

| | | |
|---|---|---|
| • chopped red onion | • crushed garlic | • sliced bell peppers |
| • sliced mushrooms | • crumbled low-fat goat or feta cheese | |
| • soy-based "pepperoni" | • blanched carrots and broccoli | |
| • fresh tomatoes | • artichoke hearts (cooked, not marinated) | |

## By the Slice

A calorie-and-fat rundown on pizza by the slice from
fast-food outlets to frozen brands.

| *Brand* | *Serving Size* | *Calories* | *Total Fat (gm)* | *Saturated Fat (gm)* |
|---|---|---|---|---|
| Domino's Cheese | 2.7 oz. slice | 190 | 5 | 3 |
| Little Caesar's Pepperoni | 3.0 oz. slice | 200 | 8 | 4 |
| Pizza Hut Pepperoni, pan | 3.7 oz. slice | 265 | 12 | 4 |
| *Frozen* | | | | |
| Healthy Choice Cheese, French bread pizza | 1 pizza | 310 | 4 | 2 |
| Lean Cuisine Cheese, French bread pizza | 1 pizza | 350 | 8 | 4 |
| Healthy Choice Pepperoni, French bread pizza | 1 pizza | 360 | 9 | 4 |
| Lean Cuisine Pepperoni, French bread pizza | 1 pizza | 330 | 7 | 3 |
| Weight Watchers Deluxe Combo | 1 entree | 380 | 11 | 3.5 |
| Lean Cuisine Deluxe, French bread pizza | 1 pizza | 330 | 6 | 2.5 |
| Healthy Choice Supreme, French bread pizza | 1 pizza | 340 | 6 | 2 |
| Healthy Choice Sausage, French bread pizza | 1 pizza | 330 | 4 | 1.5 |

*Source:* Manufacturers' Food Labels and Bowes & Church's *Food Values of Portions Commonly Used*, 17th ed., Lippincott, 1998.

mushrooms, fresh tomatoes (for more lycopene), red onions, and even crushed garlic. If it's vegetable, you can't go wrong even if it sits on top of a pizza.

If meat toppings tickle your taste buds, then ask for chicken, shrimp, or extra lean beef as toppers. When making your own, use reduced-fat or fat-free sausage. Also, try faux meat toppings made from isolated-soy protein. Soy-based sausage, pepperoni, and crumbled veggie burger can be used as tasty toppings that add the heart-healthy goodness of soy.

For more topping ideas along with assembly instructions on making your own pizza see the "Top It Off" chart on page 215. I also include my best picks on frozen pizza brands in "By the Slice" on the previous page. You can save time and your heart by topping off your frozen cheese pizza before baking with extra sliced fresh peppers, mushrooms, or onions. Just allow a few minutes of extra baking time.

# Popcorn

Movies and popcorn go together. But reports from the food-watchdogs at the Center for Science in the Public Interest have scared many movie-goers into shying away from popcorn because of its fat content. According to their reports, a large-sized movie popcorn packs over 70 grams of fat (more than a day's worth) and over 50 grams of it is artery-clogging saturated fat. But popcorn on its own is not a fat-disaster. It's when you pop it in coconut oil and top popcorn off with butter that this glorious snack becomes a heart-stopper. But without such negative adornment, popcorn is actually good for your heart.

A three-cup serving of air-popped popcorn contains a mere 90 calories, no fat, and a good dose of fiber. And the fiber in popcorn is the same cholesterol-lowering type you find in corn. Those annoying corn "shells" that get stuck in your teeth are loaded with fiber. Studies show that eating corn fiber or bran for just six weeks can lower both total cholesterol and triglyceride levels.

Making your own heart-healthy popcorn is a snap. Acquire an air-popper if popcorn is one of your dietary staples. You can liven up the flavor of plain popped corn with a sprinkle of grated Parmesan cheese, low-sodium seasoning, or fat-free butter replacement. Microwave popcorn is a convenient option that saves time and is also easy on your heart. Many brands are fat-free or have only a few grams. But watch for sodium content if you have been advised by your physician to cut back. Some brands have

## Pop Chart

How does your favorite popcorn brand stack up?

| Brands Serving = approx. 3 cups popped | Calories | Fat (gm) | Saturated Fat (gm) | Fiber (gm) | Sodium (mg) |
|---|---|---|---|---|---|
| Healthy Choice Natural | 45 | 0 | 0 | 3 | 72 |
| Pop-Secret 94% Fat-Free | 60 | 0 | 0 | 3 | 144 |
| America's Best Butter 94% Fat-Free | 50 | 1 | 0 | 5 | 130 |
| Orville Redenbacher's Smart Pop! Low-Fat | 45 | 0 | 0 | 3 | 72 |
| Orville Redenbacher's Natural Light | 60 | 2 | 0 | 3 | 72 |
| Air-popped, plain | 90 | 1 | 0.2 | 4 | 1 |
| Cracker Jack Fat-Free | 150 | 0 | 0 | 3 | 120 |
| Fiddle Faddle Fat-Free | 110 | 0 | 0 | 1 | 210 |
| Orville Redenbacher's Butter Light | 60 | 2 | 0 | 2 | 72 |
| Jolly Time Light Butter | 60 | 3 | 0 | 3 | 75 |

*Source:* Manufacturers' Food Labels and Bowes and Church's *Food Values of Portions Commonly Used,* 17th ed., Lippincott, 1998.

over 400 milligrams in a three-cup serving, while others come in under 200 milligrams.

Check out the "Pop Chart" for some of the great popcorn picks. Ready-made popcorn sold in the snack food section of your local grocery store is another good choice. Just check the label for added fat and number of fat grams per serving. Be aware that some of the cheese-flavored popcorns come with over 30 grams of fat in a three-cup serving. Also note that "air-popped" on the package label does not mean fat-free. Many manufacturers add oil or cheese to air-popped corn before packaging. Check the label to know what you are getting.

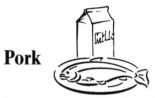

# Pork

Before you cross pork off your list of healthy foods because of bacon and pork spare ribs, take another look. Certain cuts of pork, especially tenderloin and loin chops, have less than 10 grams of fat per three-ounce serving cooked. A serving of tenderloin, for example, has a mere five grams of fat, comparable to roasted chicken served without the skin. And only one-third of the fat in pork is saturated fat. The cholesterol content of pork is also the same as an equal serving of fish or chicken. But the good news about pork is that this meat is packed with nutrients to keep your heart healthy.

A serving of pork supplies about 20 percent of your need for vitamin $B_6$. This vitamin, along with folate and vitamin $B_{12}$, helps clear the blood of a substance called *homocysteine*. Researchers now suspect that chronically elevated levels of homocysteine damage the arteries and may be a major factor in the development of heart disease. Pork also packs a good dose of zinc. Some of the enzymes that protect your cells from oxidative damage thought to cause heart disease rely on adequate levels of zinc in the diet. Many people fail to meet their need for this mineral because of poor eating habits.

Pork, like other meat, should be used in your diet a few times a week. Select leaner cuts and trim the visible fat. When cooking pork, you don't have to go to great lengths to overcook it because of food poisoning concerns. Cooking pork to an internal temperature of 160 degrees is sufficient (the same temperature guideline as beef or other meats).

Combine thin strips of pork tenderloin with several types of chopped vegetables for a tasty stir-fry. I like combining pork with beans, peppers, onions, and garlic for a fiery chili dish. Try my recipe and be sure to serve it over baked potatoes for an awesome heart-warming meal.

### *Fiery Pork and Bean Chili*

1 pound pork loin, trimmed of visible fat, cut into 3/4-inch cubes

1 yellow onion, chopped

1 bell pepper, seeded and chopped

2 tsp. chili powder

1 tsp. ground cinnamon

1 1/2 tsp. cumin

1 tsp. chili flakes or 1 hot pepper of your choice, finely chopped

2 cans kidney beans, drained

5 large tomatoes, chopped (can use 2 cans chopped tomatoes instead)

salt substitute and pepper to taste

In a large skillet with a lid, brown pork and pour off any residual fat drippings. Add onion and bell pepper, sauté a few minutes more. Then add spices, chili flakes (or hot pepper), and chopped tomatoes. Cover and let simmer 45 minutes to 1 hour. Add beans and cook another 15 minutes. Garnish with fresh coriander or green onions. Serve over cornbread or rice. Serves eight.

**Nutrition Facts**

Fiery Pork and Bean Chili

Serving Size 1/8 recipe

| Amount per Serving | |
|---|---|
| Calories 231 | 81 Calories from fat |

| | % Daily Value |
|---|---|
| Total Fat 9g | 14% |
|     Saturated Fat 3g | 15% |
| Cholesterol 60mg | 20% |
| Sodium 59mg | 2% |
| Total Carbohydrate 15g | 5% |
|     Dietary Fiber 7g | 26% |
| Protein 23g | |

| | | |
|---|---|---|
| Vitamin A 9% | • | Vitamin C 48% |
| Calcium 4% | • | Iron 10% |
| Zinc 18% | • | Vitamin B$_6$ 19% |

# Potato

A potato is what I consider one of Mother Nature's nearly perfect "packaged" foods. Classified as a tuber, the potato comes packed with an array of nutrients that help fend off heart disease and high blood pressure. One baked potato with the skin (about four inches by two and a half inches) has a hefty 900 milligram dose of potassium, over 40 percent of daily vitamin C needs, about 20 percent of fiber, and 35 percent of vitamin B$_6$, a B vitamin that helps clear the artery-damaging homocysteine from your system. All this and more comes in one potato for only 200 calories. And according to researchers who study the dietary habits of people from the Mediterranean region known for their low heart-disease risk, potatoes are a must.

Dr. Walter Willet from the Harvard School of Public Health, along with researchers from around the world, have studied the traditional diets of people from Crete, other parts of Greece, and southern Italy. Their interest is the connection between the diet and the long life expectancy and low rates of heart disease of these people. A key aspect of the Mediterranean diet is that a majority of their foods come from plants—breads, cereals, other grains, and of course, potatoes. Willet believes that the nutrients in potatoes and these other foods interact giving the body protection against heart disease. Potatoes, for example, supply ample amounts of vitamin C and fiber which both shield the arteries from cholesterol.

Other research studies with laboratory animals suggest that the protein in a potato, about five to six grams in one (a little less than what's in a glass of milk), may help lower cholesterol levels. Researchers have begun to look at what's called the amino acids profile (building blocks of protein) of various food proteins to see how this may alter the development of heart disease. When fed potato protein, cholesterol levels dropped significantly in laboratory animals compared to a protein called *casein* from dairy products. These results may help explain in part why people who eat a diet rich in potatoes have a lower risk for heart disease.

When it comes to eating potatoes, remember: The closer potatoes are to their natural state the better they are for your heart. French fries, potato chips, and dehydrated "instant" mashed potatoes have lost much of their heart-saving powers by the time they reach your plate. You're better off selecting potatoes from the produce department and then having your way with them.

There are three general categories of potatoes: new (thin-skinned reds or golds), good for salads and roasting; all purpose, good for salads, boiling, stews, and baking; and Russet potatoes, good for baking and mashing. Select potatoes free of "eyes" or sprouting; also avoid those with areas of green or large cuts or soft spots.

Store potatoes at home in a dark, cool place but not the refrigerator since typical fridge temperatures tend to be cold enough to dampen potato flavor. If your potatoes sprout or turn green during storage, be sure to cut away this portion before cooking as small amounts of a cancer-causing agent form during sprouting.

Boil them, mash them, roast them, or bake them. Do what you will to a potato but please leave the skin on for more heart-healthy nutrients. Potatoes go well in stews or casseroles, or add to soups as a hearty ingredient. When making "cream" soups, blend cooked potatoes in a food processor for a creamy texture. If you enjoy French fries, try a very low-fat, heart-healthy version: Cut oven-baking whole potatoes (with their skins on) into thin half-inch wedges and spray lightly with cooking oil spray. Bake in the oven at 375 degrees until done (about 30 minutes).

My favorite potato dish of all is creamy mashed potatoes. Leaving the skin on may at first sound gritty, but I assure you once you try mashed potatoes à la skins, you'll never go back. You can also use leftover mashed potatoes to make potato pancakes for a breakfast treat. Try out my Garlic Mashed Potatoes, packed with calcium from nonfat yogurt (used instead of cream).

### *Garlic Mashed Potatoes*

8 large Russet potatoes, washed, cut into 1 1/2-inch cubes with skin left on

5 cloves of garlic (more if you are a garlic fan)

1 1/2 cups of nonfat, plain yogurt

ground white pepper to taste

1/2 tsp. salt or salt substitute

In a large pot, boil potatoes in enough water to cover half to two-thirds of the potatoes. Toss in garlic cloves when potatoes are almost done (last five minutes of cooking). When soft enough to mash, drain potatoes and garlic. Mash with a potato masher, large fork, or hand mixer (a mixer makes creamier mashed potatoes). Add yogurt, pepper to taste, and salt or salt substitute. Serves eight to ten.

**Nutrition Facts**

Garlic Mashed Potatoes

Serving Size 1/10 recipe

| Amount per Serving | |
|---|---|
| Calories 246 | 0 Calories from fat |

| | % Daily Value |
|---|---|
| Total Fat 0g | 0% |
| Saturated Fat 0g | 0% |
| Cholesterol 0mg | 0% |
| Sodium 182mg | 8% |
| Total Carbohydrate 55g | 18% |
| Dietary Fiber 5g | 19% |
| Protein 7g | |

| | | |
|---|---|---|
| Vitamin A 0% | • | Vitamin C 45% |
| Calcium 11% | • | Iron 16% |

# Prunes

When I munch on a handful of prunes, I think of my grandmother. She touted their benefits swearing that eating prunes daily was good for what ails you. I believed her. But I always figured she meant they were good for relieving constipation (prunes and prune juice contain a substance that has a laxative effect). Years later I know that eating prunes every day may also keep the doctor away by lowering blood cholesterol levels.

Made from a special variety of plum best suited for drying, prunes are packed with fiber. A serving of 10 prunes has about six grams of fiber and most of it is pectin, a type of water-soluble fiber that helps lower blood cholesterol. Once inside your intestinal tract, pectin latches on to cholesterol from foods or bile (a substance in your intestinal tract made from cholesterol) and keeps cholesterol from getting into your circulation.

Researchers from the University of California, Davis Nutrition Department demonstrated that a daily intake of prunes is an effective way to lower blood cholesterol levels. Study participants with already high cholesterol levels were asked to eat about 12 prunes daily for eight weeks. Compared to when the same subjects drank grape juice as a control, levels of LDLs, the artery-damaging carrier of cholesterol, fell significantly.

There is something else about prunes you might want to know. Blended with water into a puree, prunes can be used as a replacement for fat. Use it just like applesauce; add prune puree to cakes, muffins, and cookies in place of butter or margarine, and you will lower the fat and calorie content dramatically (not to mention adding heart-healthy fiber). Make the puree in a blender or food processor by adding four ounces of pitted prunes with five tablespoons of water. Or you can also save time and purchase prune purée sold at your local supermarket. Sunsweet® makes a product called "Lighter Bake" which can be used as a fat replacement in baked goods such as cookies, muffins, and cakes. Try my spiced carrot cake recipe, and you'll be surprised how moist and rich it tastes.

You can use whole or chopped prunes in many ways—as a topping for cereal (hot or cold), yogurt, cottage cheese, or low-fat ice cream; or add prunes to a fresh fruit salad for extra fiber. I like to add chopped prunes to my morning smoothie for a rich texture.

### *Carrot Cake sans Fat*

3/4 cup prune puree or Lighter Bake® from Sunsweet

3/4 cup each of white and brown sugar

4 egg whites or 1/2 cup egg substitute

2 tsp. vanilla

2 1/4 cups flour

2 tsp. baking soda

2 tsp. cinnamon

3/4 tsp. nutmeg

1/4 tsp. cloves

3 cups grated carrots (use a food processor)

1 cup raisins

3/4 cup chopped walnuts (optional)

In a large bowl, beat sugars, prune puree, egg whites, and vanilla until light. Combine dry ingredients in another bowl. Stir dry ingredients into prune-egg mixture. Then add carrots and raisins (walnuts if desired). Spread batter into a 13 x 9-inch baking pan sprayed with cooking spray. Bake at 375 degrees for 30 to 40 minutes or until an inserted toothpick comes out clean. Cool and dust with powdered sugar, or garnish with a dollop of nonfat vanilla frozen yogurt. Makes 12 servings.

| **Nutrition Facts** | |
| :--- | ---: |
| Carrot Cake sans Fat | |
| Serving Size 1/12 recipe | |
| **Amount per Serving** | |
| Calories 328      40 Calories from fat | |
| | % Daily Value |
| Total Fat 5g | 7% |
| Saturated Fat <.5g | 2% |
| Cholesterol 0mg | 0% |
| Sodium 176mg | 7% |
| Total Carbohydrate 68g | 23% |
| Dietary Fiber 3g | 11% |
| Protein 6g | |
| Vitamin A 90%  •  Vitamin C 6% | |
| Calcium 4%  •  Iron 13% | |

# Pumpkin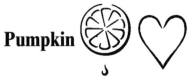

Despite pumpkin's seasonal appearance at Halloween and Thanksgiving, this fruit should make a regular appearance in your diet to keep heart disease and hypertension at bay. (Pumpkin is a fruit, not a vegetable, since it is a member of the gourd family like melons.) Pumpkin is packed with a staggering 10,000 milligrams of a mixture of carotenes in a half-cup serving of cooked, mashed pumpkin. Carotenes, such as beta and alpha carotene, are bright orange plant pigments that give pumpkin and other fruits and vegetables their characteristic color. And it's the mixture of carotenes along with the fiber and potassium in pumpkin that keep your heart healthy.

Studies show that both a potassium-rich and fiber-filled diet help lower blood pressure, and pumpkin does both. Each serving of pumpkin contains almost 300 milligrams of potassium or about 10 percent of your daily needs, along with about 4 grams of fiber or 20 percent of your daily need. The carotenes in pumpkins are antioxidants. Both beta and alpha carotene help protect cells from damage caused by dangerous molecules called *free radicals*. The LDLs, which carry cholesterol throughout the body, are protected from free radical damage by powerful carotene antioxidants.

Pumpkin-enriched fare may also help lower cholesterol levels. Preliminary studies with laboratory animals show that adding pumpkin to their daily diets significantly lowers blood cholesterol levels. This is positive news considering that these animals were fed fatty diets designed to purposely elevate their cholesterol levels.

But are you willing to carve a whole pumpkin, bake it in the oven or microwave, and then mash it up for eating? You and I don't have the time. And since fresh pumpkins only make a brief appearance at your grocery store during the month of October, reach for canned pumpkin any time of year. In fact, canned pumpkin is richer in carotenes than fresh because the canned version has less water which results in a greater nutrient density.

Pumpkin is traditionally used in desserts—pies, muffins, dessert breads, and even cookies. Try my pumpkin pie recipe; it doesn't have to be holiday time to enjoy this power-packed treat. But this versatile fruit works well in other dishes, too. Use mashed pumpkin as you would a winter squash. Season with herbs and use as a side dish, or combine with cooked potatoes and serve as "orange mashed pumptatoes." Pumpkin soup made with vegetable broth is a heart warming dish, especially on a cold winter day.

## Anytime Pumpkin Pie

Single pie crust (ready-made type or make your own using canola oil and *trans*–fat free margarine in place of shortening or butter)

1 10-oz. can of mashed pumpkin

1/4 cup egg substitute

1 can evaporated skim milk

1/3 cup brown sugar

1 tsp. cinnamon

1/2 tsp. cloves

1/4 tsp. ginger

1/4 tsp. nutmeg

Mix all ingredients (except pie crust) in a large bowl with a wire whisk. Pour into the unbaked pie crust. Bake at 425 degrees for 15 minutes and turn oven down to 350 degrees for a remaining 30 minutes. Let cool before serving. Top with vanilla flavored low-fat or nonfat yogurt, or a reduced-fat whipped topping. Makes eight servings.

## Nutrition Facts

Anytime Pumpkin Pie
Serving Size 1/8 of pie

| Amount per Serving | |
|---|---|
| Calories 196      67 Calories from fat | |
| | % Daily Value |
| Total Fat 7g | 12% |
| Saturated Fat 3g | 16% |
| Cholesterol 6mg | 2% |
| Sodium 151mg | 6% |
| Total Carbohydrate 28g | 9% |
| Dietary Fiber 1g | 3% |
| Protein 4g | |

Vitamin A 95%  •  Vitamin C 3%
Calcium 11%  •  Iron 7%

# Rhubarb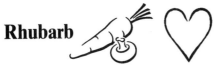

In ancient Greek times, rhubarb was referred to as the "vegetable of the barbarians." Perhaps rhubarb, which consists of celery-like stalks, earned this title because of its tart, almost bitter taste. And the leaves of rhubarb, not recommended for eating, contain a toxin that if eaten in large enough amounts is poisonous. Despite rhubarb's bad rap, this vegetable—which is actually used as a fruit in pies, tarts, and preserves—is good for your heart. Rhubarb's nutritional profile is nothing to boast about: 26 calories per cup with a dose of vitamin C and calcium along with 10 percent of your fiber needs. But it's the special fiber in rhubarb that may work wonders on your blood cholesterol levels.

Through his laboratory work, Dr. Vinti Goel from the University of Alberta in Edmonton, Canada, found strong evidence of rhubarb's special heart-healthy powers. A group of men with risky levels of blood cholesterol were fed about an ounce of rhubarb fiber daily for four weeks. (The rhubarb fiber was made from drying out stalks and grinding to a powder.) At the end of the four weeks, blood cholesterol dropped significantly from previous levels and LDL, the bad carrier of cholesterol, also dropped substantially. All this with no change in HDL levels, the good cholesterol carrier that helps lower heart-disease risk.

Adding rhubarb to your diet takes a sweet touch. Because of its bitterness, some sweetener must be added when cooking rhubarb. Start with fresh crisp stalks or purchase frozen, chopped rhubarb that has just as much fiber as fresh. Use rhubarb as you would apples or other fruits that can be baked or cooked until soft. Sweeten to taste with a mixture of brown sugar and molasses for extra nutrition. I like baking rhubarb with apples and raisins in a "crisp" for a heart-smart dessert. It's great served warm and topped with a small scoop of vanilla fat-free frozen yogurt. Here's a different type of rhubarb recipe in a curry dish. This curry is a bit spicy and sour, but quite tasty.

## *Rhubarb Curry with Catfish*

2 cups rhubarb, chopped (1/2 inch)

1 large yellow onion, chopped

1 tbsp. fresh ginger, chopped

1/2 tsp. turmeric

1/2 tsp. powdered chili or chili flakes

1/2 tsp. paprika

5 large tomatoes, chopped

1/2 bunch of fresh coriander, chopped (garnish)

4 tbsp. olive oil

4 catfish fillets (1 1/2 to 2 lb.)

Heat oil in skillet and sauté rhubarb, onion, and ginger until soft. Add spices and tomatoes. Cook until tomatoes are soft. Add fish, covering with tomato mixture. Cover skillet and cook until fish is done, about 10 to 15 minutes. Garnish with fresh chopped coriander and serve over hot rice. Makes six to seven servings.

| **Nutrition Facts** | |
|---|---|
| Rhubarb Curry with Catfish | |
| Serving Size 1/7 recipe | |
| Amount per Serving | |
| Calories 251    126 Calories from fat | |
| | % Daily Value |
| Total Fat 14g | 22% |
| Saturated Fat 2g | 12% |
| Cholesterol 66mg | 22% |
| Sodium 86mg | 4% |
| Total Carbohydrate 9g | 3% |
| Dietary Fiber 3g | 11% |
| Protein 22g | |
| Vitamin A 11%  •  Vitamin C 40% | |
| Calcium 9%  •  Iron 10% | |
| Vitamin E 29%  •  Vitamin $B_{12}$ 42% | |

# Rice

Along with olive oil and red wine, rice is on the list of traditional dietary staples of the Mediterranean. And since eating a Mediterranean-style diet may cut your heart-disease risk, rice is a must in your Simple Six Eating Plan. Packed with a bounty of carbohydrates, vitamins, and special cholesterol busters, rice will make a heart-healthy foundation to almost any meal.

The outer covering or bran layer from a grain of brown or wild rice contains substances proven to lower blood cholesterol levels. (White rice lacks this outer bran layer which is removed during processing.) These powerful substances are called *oryzanol* and *tocotrienols,* and are found in the oil from rice bran. They have been shown to significantly lower blood cholesterol levels. Researchers believe these substances may block cholesterol production in the body much the same way some prescription-only, cholesterol-lowering drugs work.

According to a study from LSU in Baton Rouge, Louisiana, adding rice bran to your diet (either as brown or wild rice, or as rice bran) may assist in your crusade against heart disease. Subjects with dangerous levels of blood cholesterol were chosen to be in this study. A group of subjects ate a rice-bran enriched diet (about three ounces daily) for three weeks. By the end of the three short weeks, the rice-bran treatment resulted in significant drops in both total cholesterol and artery-clogging LDL cholesterol.

Rice bran was a helpful addition to Ed's diet. His cholesterol levels dropped 10 percent. Since Ed's food allergy to wheat kept him from eating many standard whole-grain products, I suggested he give rice bran a try. He welcomed the opportunity to add rice bran to his meals (added to hot cereal, soups, and more) and with great success!

Besides cholesterol-lowering oryzanol and tocotrienols in rice bran, other heart-healthy nutrients abound. Both brown and wild rice provide a dose of vitamin $B_6$, along with two other B vitamins, folate and B$_{12}$, crucial in keeping circulating levels of homocysteine in check (the amino acid metabolite linked to heart disease). Rice bran and brown rice also supply a decent amount of vitamin E, known to protect against heart disease, with just over 10 percent of your needs in a one-cup serving.

Rice is one of those heart-healthy standby foods you should always have on hand—it's inexpensive, stores well, and cooks up in a short time, ready to enhance any meal. If you buy rice in bulk, make sure to keep it stored in an airtight container in your pantry.

Selecting a rice to meet your needs can be tricky, though, when you take a look at all the possibilities. Most rice varieties vary by grain length. Long grain rice is desired for its fluffy texture that stays separate or "flaky"—great for pilafs, curries, and as a cradle for stir-fries and other toppings. Shorter grains cook up moister and tend to stick together, making them ideal for rice ball appetizers and sushi, and also for smothering with steamed vegetables and the like. If you want to make risotto (Italian rice-broth dish), use ariborio or carnaroli rice, which both develop a creamy texture during cooking (crucial for a good risotto) when patiently stirred. If you try my creamy Portobello Mushroom Risotto recipe on page 187, it will become a popular main dish in your home, too.

There is an endless number of ways to use rice. Start your day out with chilled cooked brown rice (maybe leftover from the day before) and top it with nonfat milk, and a handful of raisins and walnuts for more heart-healthy nutrition. Open a can of ready-to-eat soup and add cooked rice, heat through and you have a great bowl of soup. Make up a chilled rice salad with your favorite chopped vegetables and serve as a side dish, or add cooked black beans and make a meal of it. Try my Rice-Lentil Salad loaded with cholesterol-lowering fiber.

One of my favorite ways to use rice is as a stuffing for baked vegetables—eggplant, winter squash, or tomato. Just season rice with fresh herbs, onion, or garlic, stir in some vegetable broth, then you're ready to stuff a whole vegetable (make a hole by removing the seeds). Bake for about an hour, serve with some mixed greens and you have a delicious heart-healthy meal.

## Rice-Lentil Salad

2 cups cooked brown rice
1 can lentils, drained or 1 1/2 cups cooked lentils
1/2 cucumber, diced
1 carrot, diced
1 tomato, chopped
3 scallions, chopped
1/4 cup parsley, chopped
3 tbsp. seasoned rice vinegar
1 tsp. sesame oil
1 tsp. prepared mustard, Dijon style
juice from half a lemon

In a large bowl, combine rice, lentils, cucumber, tomato, scallions, and parsley. In a small jar with a tight fitting lid, combine vinegar, oil, mustard, and lemon juice and shake well. Pour over rice mixture and toss well. Chill at least an hour before serving. Makes about five one-cup servings.

| **Nutrition Facts** | |
|---|---|
| Rice-Lentil Salad | |
| Serving Size 1 cup | |
| Amount per Serving | |
| Calories 184        18 Calories from fat | |
| | % Daily Value |
| Total Fat 2g | 3% |
| Saturated Fat 0g | 0% |
| Cholesterol 0mg | 0% |
| Sodium 28mg | 1% |
| Total Carbohydrate 35g | 12% |
| Dietary Fiber 6g | 23% |
| Protein 8g | |
| Vitamin A 50%  •  Vitamin C 22% | |
| Calcium 4%  •  Iron 16% | |

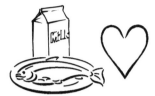

# Salmon

Salmon is truly the king when it comes to netting the heart-healthy benefits of fish. At first glance though, salmon's stats may look daunting: Each three-ounce serving contains over nine grams of fat or almost half of the total calories. But the fat in salmon, as with other fatty fish, is heart-healthy. Very little of the fat is the saturated, artery-clogging version, while most of the fat is mononounsaturated which studies show helps lower blood cholesterol. Also, salmon is a source of omega-3 fats, a type of polyunsaturated fat that works wonders on your heart. Each serving has just over a gram of omega-3 and according to research, regular servings of fish like salmon cut the risk of heart attacks and sudden death from heart attacks.

A group of researchers from Bringham Women's Hospital and Harvard Medical School in Massachusetts studied the eating habits and heart health of over 20,000 men for almost 11 years. During this time, there were over 130 sudden deaths from heart attacks. The researchers found that those men who consumed a three- to four-ounce serving of fish at least once a week had half the risk of dying from a sudden heart attack compared to men who consumed no fish.

Scientists believe that omega-3 fats, a very "fluid" or "squishy" type of fat, become incorporated into the cells of heart tissue, which in turn helps lessen the risk for abnormal heartbeats. As part of the cell structure, omega-3s also help modulate the flow of calcium and other substances crucial for regular heartbeats. Arrhythmias, irregular or abnormal heartbeats, contribute to sudden death following a heart attack.

In another study, this time in Italy, home of the Mediterranean diet, women were found to have 40 percent less risk of acute heart attack if fish was a regular part of their diet. Besides lowering blood fat levels, omega-3 fats keep blood cells from clumping together. This helps minimize sudden blood clots from forming and blocking off arteries that feed the heart muscle with much needed oxygen.

Besides omega-3s, salmon has even more heart-saving goodness. Each three-ounce serving supplies over 200 percent of vitamin $B_{12}$ needs. This B vitamin helps keep circulating levels of homocysteine in check, the ravaging menace of blood vessels, thus lessening heart disease progression. And if you eat canned salmon with the fine, virtually-undetectable bones, you get a hefty 200 plus milligrams of calcium, which may help to lower blood pressure.

## Go Fishing

So what's keeping you from eating salmon, or other fish on a more regular basis? If you're like most, you may shy away from eating fish because you find yourself treading in unfamiliar waters. Use these simple guidelines in selecting, storing, and preparing fresh fish properly.

- *Shop at reputable fish markets.* Ask when fish was caught or brought into the store. All fish should be displayed on ice.
- *Smell fish for signs of freshness.* Fresh fish should not have a "fishy" odor.
- *Store fish in your refrigerator and plan on using it within a day.* Unlike chicken, beef, and other meats, fish starts to decay even when refrigerated within about two to three days—you will be able to tell by the fishy odor.
- *If you freeze fresh fish, wrap it in freezer paper and date it.* Use within about three months.
- *Thaw fish in your refrigerator* for about two to three hours, or for thin fish fillets, cook frozen and just add to the cooking time.
- *Cook fish in a baking dish, in aluminum foil, or on a rack with few holes or grid lines.* Fish tends to break apart easily during cooking with the exception of firmer fish such as swordfish and shark, which makes these ideal for grilling.

- *Knowing when fish is "done" can be perplexing.* Properly cooked fish flakes apart with a fork. All fish should be cooked to 145 degrees for about five minutes. This takes about 10 to 13 minutes per inch of fish (thickness). Best baking temperature for fish is 425 to 450 degrees.

- *Broiling fish typically requires less cooking time* because of higher temperatures. Thick fillets should be turned using about four to six minutes per side.

- *Microwaving or poaching fish requires adding some liquid such as vegetable broth or wine.* Use the same "flaking" test for doneness, and follow microwave manufacturer's instructions for cooking fish.

- *Grill fish either directly on the grill (firm fish) or wrap in foil* with lemon slices and herbs such as dill or rosemary and cook until done.

My favorite way to prepare fresh salmon fillets is wrapped in foil with sprigs of fresh herbs, a touch of wine, and ground pepper sprinkled on top. I either bake this in an oven (done in less than 15 minutes at 425 degrees), or if I'm in the mood, I place this package directly on the grill along with kabobs of fresh vegetables (peppers, cherry tomatoes, onions). Served with crusty sourdough whole-wheat bread and a glass of wine, this is my idea of a perfect weekend meal.

### *Miso-Marinated Salmon*

Miso Marinade (see page 183 for recipe)
5 fresh salmon fillets (five servings or about 1 1/2 pounds)

In a glass baking dish, marinate salmon fillets for 30 minutes. Grill or broil salmon for 10 minutes (depending on fillet thickness) until done (flaky inside). Serve with lemon and fresh chopped coriander as garnish. Serves five.

**Nutrition Facts**

Miso-Marinated Salmon

Serving Size 1 fillet (1/5 recipe)

| Amount per Serving | |
| --- | --- |
| Calories 287      126 Calories from fat | |
| | % Daily Value |
| Total Fat 14g | 22% |
| Saturated Fat 3g | 17% |
| Cholesterol 90mg | 30% |
| Sodium 191mg | 8% |
| Total Carbohydrate 9g | 3% |
| Dietary Fiber <1g | 1% |
| Protein 28g | |

| | | |
| --- | --- | --- |
| Vitamin A 21% | • | Vitamin C 10% |
| Calcium 3% | • | Iron 6% |
| Vitamin E 20% | • | Vitamin $B_{12}$ 68% |

# Salsa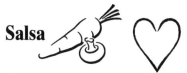

Move over catsup, salsa is here, and in a big way. What's haute these days is hot. Salsa, the Mexican word for sauce, is typically a combination of mild to hot chilies, onions, garlic, tomatoes, and even fruit. These days, you'll find salsas topping everything from morning scrambled eggs and potatoes to evening meatloaf and potatoes. And what better way to spice up your meals and at the same time protect your heart? Salsa, especially if you make up your own, is a powerhouse of heart-saving vitamins, minerals, and phytochemicals that can help stave off high blood pressure, lower blood cholesterol levels, and keep arteries from clogging.

Salsa comes in three basic types: a cooked version usually made with tomato, onion, garlic, pepper, and chili of some sort; a fresh variety typically a combination of the same ingredients along with cilantro (fragrant Mexican parsley), and lime juice; and a fruit salsa often made with papaya, mango, citrus fruit, pineapple, or any type of fresh fruit you desire with onions, cilantro, and chilies (you get the idea).

All of these ingredients in salsa act like an orchestra of powerful substances that together bring you the harmony of heart health. Depending on the style of salsa, you get a dose of vitamin C from tomato, onion, and peppers that helps protect LDLs from becoming damaging to artery walls. You get the heart-saving benefits of the many phytochemicals from garlic, onions, hot peppers, tomatoes, cilantro, and fruit. And to top it off, if you like to pile on the salsa, you also get a good dose of cholesterol-lowering soluble fiber.

You can easily purchase heart-healthy salsa. Bottled or jarred salsas are of the cooked variety. Watch for added fats in some brands and unwanted sodium if you need to restrict your intake on the advice of a physician. You can find fresh salsas in the refrigerator section of your grocery store. Restaurants serve tomato-based salsas and sometimes fresh fruit salsas, which go especially well with grilled fish or poultry. Oftentimes, Mexican-style eateries have salsa "bars" featuring several types of salsas—from cooked to fresh, mild to spicy hot, so take your pick.

I prefer to make my own salsa. It takes a matter of seconds and this way I know everything is fresh and at its peak of heart-healthy nutrition. All it takes to make a great salsa is fresh ingredients and a small food processor. Keep on hand tomatoes, garlic, cilantro, red onion, hot peppers of your choice, and anything else you like in your salsa. Simply whir the ingredients in the food processor using the pulse feature to allow a chopping action. And ta-da! You have fresh salsa. Yes, on occasion I do make cooked salsa. This, of course, takes extra time that many of us have little of. That's okay, though, since fresh salsa is packed with more heart-healthy nutrients than cooked because heat destroys some of the heart-healthy goodies.

You can dip, slather, smother, or otherwise drown anything in salsa. It's up to your taste buds. And since salsa is fat-free (check the label if using commercial varieties), and loaded with nutrients, you are better off with gobs of salsa than even small dabs of creamy sauces and dips that can be dangerous to your heart. Try my recipe for Cantaloupe Salsa; it makes a wonderful addition to grilled fish. As an added bonus, the cantaloupe supplies heart-protecting carotenes.

## Cantaloupe Salsa

1 large cantaloupe, seeded and chopped into small pieces

1 small red onion, chopped fine

1 hot pepper (jalapeño), chopped very fine (may want to use a food processor)

1/4 cup chopped coriander

juice from 2 limes

4 large tomatoes, chopped

In a large bowl, mix all ingredients together. Chill at least a half hour before serving. Makes about eight servings.

| **Nutrition Facts** | |
| --- | --- |
| Cantaloupe Salsa | |
| Serving Size 1/8 recipe | |
| Amount per Serving | |
| Calories 42 | 0 Calories from fat |
| | % Daily Value |
| Total Fat 0g | 0% |
| Saturated Fat 0g | 0% |
| Cholesterol 0mg | 0% |
| Sodium 28mg | 1% |
| Total Carbohydrate 10g | 3% |
| Dietary Fiber 2g | 6% |
| Protein 1g | |
| Vitamin A 29% • Vitamin C 70% | |
| Calcium 1% • Iron 3% | |
| • Potassium 10% | |

# Salt Sense

Salty chips, lip-smacking French fries, crunchy pretzels, and addictive popcorn—these all taste great thanks to salt, one of those flavors we just can't seem to live without. Our penchant for salt started thousands of years ago when preserving food was a must for survival. Back then, salt was rare, hard to get, even used as a form of money (the word *salary* comes from the word *salt*). But today we're awash in salt. We average about two to three full teaspoons of salt daily. This supplies over 10 times our requirement for sodium, a mineral crucial to help control body fluid balance and nerve function.

But all that is salty is not good. As the research story goes, too much sodium or salt may spell trouble for blood pressure. Countless scientific studies suggest that the higher the salt intake, the greater the risk of developing hypertension, the number one risk factor for stroke. And if salt intake is reduced, blood pressure readings fall. But before you strike salt from your diet (which would be next to impossible, I might add), you should know that not everyone benefits from cutting back on the salty stuff.

For starters, only 20 percent of the population is "salt sensitive," meaning that blood pressure responds to changes in salt or sodium intake. Instead, most people's blood pressure readings reflect other factors such as body weight. Being overweight, for example, is a major cause of hypertension rather than too much salt in the diet. The only way you would know if you are salt sensitive is by trial and error, experimenting with your salt intake while at the same time obtaining blood pressure readings.

Since the search for salt sensitivity may not be practical for most, it's best to use some salt sense when it comes to seeking healthy blood pressure. A teaspoon of salt, or 2400 milligrams of sodium, daily is recommended. This represents less than half of what most Americans eat and just a fraction of what some people take in that are heavy users of catsup, soy sauce, and other salty condiments. For example, Jim, who came to me perplexed about his persistently high blood pressure readings, insisted he skimped on sodium. He was shocked to find out his average daily intake topped 4000 milligrams because of his penchant for a heavily salted brand of salsa that he poured over almost everything he ate.

The 2400 milligram limit is designed to be healthy for people with and without high blood pressure. Those with hypertension should seek the advice of their physician for use of necessary medications or diet modifications to lower blood pressure. For some individuals, cutting back on sodium along with proper medication puts blood pressure readings into the safe range.

Even though millions of Americans don't have high blood pressure, the chance hypertension will develop is almost a guarantee since risk goes up with age. So cutting back on salt now is prudent advice. Heavy use of the saltshaker or eating a diet rich in processed foods including chips, crackers, baked goods, and frozen dinners, besides threatening your heart may also cause other problems. With a diet like this, chances are there is not much room for fresh fruits and vegetables loaded with vitamins and minerals needed for healthy blood pressure readings. Also, studies show that a high sodium intake may boost the loss of calcium from the body, setting you up for bone disease later in life.

When you follow the Simple Six Eating Plan you receive plenty of minerals such as potassium and calcium, fiber, and other nutrients helpful in maintaining a healthy set of blood pressure numbers. You do not have to count milligrams of sodium you eat each day but rather enjoy more naturally low sodium foods. Eating eight to ten servings of fruits and vegetables daily adds virtually no sodium. If your physician has recommended a specific, reduced level of sodium, then follow that advice using the food labels to identify sodium content of foods.

If you know you are a salt addict, then try backing off on sodium gradually through eating more naturally low-sodium vegetables, fruits, grains, and other low-sodium foods. It takes about two months to readjust your taste preference to lower levels. Once you have adjusted, you will be surprised when you bite into a salty French fry and most likely it won't taste good to you—too salty.

There are many reduced-salt or salt-free flavoring agents you can use to liven up your foods the way salt enhances a food's flavor. You can use lemon juice or vinegar to get this same effect.

Also try salt replacements (usually made with potassium) in cooking and seasoning foods.

**Sardines**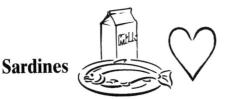

Sardines are so named because these small silvery fish were first harvested off the small Mediterranean island of Sardinia. Actually a member of the herring family, sardines come packed with a trio of stellar heart-healthy nutrients that will help fend off both hypertension and heart disease. A two-ounce serving of sardines (about four whole fish) supplies a whopping 400 percent of vitamin $B_{12}$ needs, almost 20 percent of your daily calcium requirement and a good dose of heart-healthy omega-3 fats, all for just 100 calories.

Vitamin $B_{12}$, along with folate and vitamin $B_6$, work together in clearing the bad blood factor called homocysteine that causes damage to artery walls. The hefty dose of $B_{12}$ in a serving of sardines is good news since many people skimp on other major sources, such as beef and eggs. The calcium in sardines works in modulating blood pressure. Studies show that people who consume calcium-rich foods like dairy products and sardines have a lower risk for hypertension than those who fall short on calcium needs.

The omega-3 fats in sardines, as in other seafood, protect your heart in several ways. Eating one to two servings of fish weekly has been shown to cut the risk of death from heart attacks. Studies show that the omega-3 fats in sardines and other fatty fish, such as salmon, keep blood cells from sticking or clumping together. This anticlumping action will help avoid a deadly heart attack or stroke. In addition, fish fat has been shown to lower high blood pressure, particularly in people with mild hypertension. (Check out the "Gone Fishing" chart on omega-3s in fish.)

Virtually all sardines sold in the U.S. are canned, so look for sardines next to canned tuna and clams in your grocery store. If you can find sardines packed in fish oil, snatch them up as you'll

## Gone Fishing

Eating one serving of fish weekly may cut your risk of suffering from a fatal heart attack. To help you select omega-3 powerhouses, use this listing for three-ounces of fresh fish and other seafood.

| *Best* (more than 1 gm) | *Better* (0.5 to 1.0 gm) | *Good* (less than 0.5 gm) |
|---|---|---|
| Anchovy | Albacore tuna, canned | Catfish |
| Bluefin tuna | Bass | Clams |
| Carp | Halibut | Cod |
| Herring | Oyster | Crab |
| Mackerel | Pollock | Flounder |
| Salmon | Rainbow trout | Haddock |
| Sardines | Rock fish | Lobster |
| Sturgeon | Shark | Perch |
| | Smelt | Scallops |
| | | Shrimp |
| | | Snapper |
| | | Sole |
| | | Squid |
| | | Swordfish |

get even more omega-3s. Sardines are more commonly sold in vegetable oil and tomato or curry sauce. Use sardines as you would other canned seafood. Mix sardines into cold pasta or green salads. Or for a change of pace, use sardines in place of canned tuna in your next sandwich.

# Sea Vegetables (a.k.a. seaweed)

Before you say "yuck," sea vegetables—better known as seaweed—makes an exotic-tasting, heart-healthy addition to your diet. Legend has it that the Greek goddess Aphrodite owed her beauty to her penchant for seaweed. (Come to think of it, mermaids must be munching on seaweed, too!) Today there are a wide variety of seaweeds used in Asian cooking that add a nutritional punch to foods. Nori, for example, a seaweed traditionally used in making sushi and other wrapped rice appetizers, is loaded with the B vitamin folate and a good dose of calcium. Wakame, a seaweed used in soups, salads, and even sandwiches, also supplies folate—almost 50 percent of your needs in only a 45-calorie serving (3 1/2 ounces raw). And according to research studies, eating a diet with adequate folate may help fend off heart disease.

The folate/heart disease connection centers around an amino acid found in the circulation called *homocysteine*. Researchers have noted that individuals with high circulating levels of homocysteine have a greater risk of developing heart disease. It appears that homocysteine damages artery walls and accelerates the clogging of arteries. Folate's connection is with the process of breaking down homocysteine. People with low circulating levels of folate have higher homocysteine levels and vice versa; the higher the levels of folate, the lower the levels of homocysteine, and the healthier your heart will be.

Dr. Killian Robinson from the Cleveland Clinic Foundation, along with researchers from Europe, studied 700 patients with heart disease and another 800 people with no signs of heart disease. Blood samples were analyzed for homocysteine levels along with measurements taken for folate. Those individuals with the lowest levels of folate had greater circulating levels of homocysteine and a greater risk of heart disease.

Many people fall short of meeting their 400 microgram daily requirement. The best food sources of folate include green leafy vegetables such as kale and spinach, fortified breakfast cereals, and citrus fruits. However, the big standout as the abundant provider of natural folate is seaweed. You can easily meet your folate needs by including seaweed, along with other foods, in your daily fare.

Shop for seaweed at specialty Asian food stores or health food stores. In urban areas, many big grocery stores have Asian food sections that carry a variety of seaweed. Types include nori, dulse, and arame. Usually sold dry in airtight packages, seaweed should be rinsed in water before use to remove any salt crystals or small bits of shells, except for nori. Sold in sheets and already roasted, nori can be used as is for wrapping when making California rolls (check out my recipe using heart-healthy ginger and asparagus), sushi, and other dishes.

After rinsing, soak seaweed in water until it feels supple or soft. At this point, you can add chopped dulse seaweed to soups for a spicy flavor, or for a mild "ocean" flavor, use arame seaweed. Add the seaweed during the last few minutes of cooking; overcooking seaweed changes its texture. Sauté arame along with other vegetables in a stir-fry or add to cold salads (works well with cabbage and water chestnuts).

## *"Davis" California Rolls*

*I bring these as appetizers to parties—a hit every time!*

3 cups short-grain rice (Cook in 3 cups of water. When all the water is taken up, add 1 cup seasoned rice vinegar.)

1/2 cup pickled ginger (Asian market or section in grocery store)

3/4 lb. or one bunch of asparagus, steamed

1/2 cup sesame seeds

1/4 cup Japanese bonito flakes with seaweed (available at Asian markets)

1 package of roasted seaweed sheets (nori)

Set up ingredients for assembly of rolls. Place one sheet of seaweed on a flat surface. Spread cooked rice evenly over seaweed. In the center, place asparagus spears (lay across center forming a line), sprinkle one teaspoon each of sesame seeds and bonito flakes across the center (alongside asparagus). Then follow with ginger. Roll up; asparagus will be in the center of the roll as a "filling." Repeat for remaining sheets of seaweed. Wrap each roll in plastic wrap and chill at least 30 minutes. To serve, slice each roll into one-inch slices and serve with hot dipping sauce (chili paste mixed with rice vinegar works well—cool off with some iced tea!). Makes 12 servings.

| Nutrition Facts | |
| --- | --- |
| "Davis" California Rolls | |
| Serving Size 1/12 recipe | |
| **Amount per Serving** | |
| Calories 243      27 Calories from fat | |
| | % Daily Value |
| Total Fat 3g | 5% |
| Saturated Fat <1g | 3% |
| Cholesterol 0mg | 0% |
| Sodium 410mg | 17% |
| Total Carbohydrate 48g | 16% |
| Dietary Fiber 2g | 6% |
| Protein 6g | |
| Vitamin A 6%   •   Vitamin C 18% | |
| Calcium 8%   •   Iron 18% | |
| •   Folate 11% | |

# Shrimp

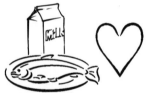

With over half your daily allotment for cholesterol in just one three-ounce serving, you might think that shrimp should rarely be a guest for dinner. Think again. Shrimp, second only to tuna in seafood popularity, is a heart-healthy food easily fitting into the Simple Six Eating Plan. Each serving provides about 20 percent of your protein needs, less than a gram of fat, and a good dose of the minerals iron and zinc in a little over 100 calories.

And to top things off, each serving of shrimp packs over 20 percent of your vitamin $B_{12}$ needs. This B vitamin, along with folate and vitamin $B_6$, plays a crucial role in clearing homocysteine from the blood, an amino-acid metabolite that, when present in high circulating levels, damages artery walls leading to heart disease.

Many of the people I work with begin their crusade against heart disease by cutting out shrimp and other seafood from their diets for fear of the cholesterol. I encourage them to eat this seafood delicacy. And here is plenty of proof: A group of researchers from Rockefeller University in New York put a group of subjects on a high shrimp diet. Each day, participants ate 11 ounces of shrimp, which put their total cholesterol intake at close to 600 milligrams, twice the recommended daily budget. Despite this cholesterol load, there was no ill effect on blood cholesterol levels and triglyceride levels (circulating fat in the blood) fell 13 percent compared to a no-shrimp, low-cholesterol diet.

Unless you live along the coast and are fortunate enough to pick up truly fresh shrimp, all shrimp sold in grocery stores and fish markets has already been frozen. Since shrimp easily spoils, freezing is a must as is spraying shrimp with sulfites soon after harvesting which help prevent the shrimp from browning.

After purchasing, plan on using shrimp within a day or two unless they are still frozen. While there are many varieties of shrimp, the only difference is their size. Small shrimp are best cooked and then chilled for use in fresh green salads or cold pasta salads. Larger shrimp make great appetizers chilled, or grilled and used in fajitas and hot pasta dishes. Cook shrimp by stir frying quickly in a nonstick pan. They turn pink when done—avoid overcooking as shrimp get tough with prolonged heating.

In place of chicken, beef, or other seafood, try shrimp. They are especially wonderful in stir-fry dishes with plenty of quick-cooked bell peppers and snow peas. Try jumbo shrimp in a seafood stew, or marinate in lime juice, garlic, and soy sauce. Grill and serve with risotto along with a mixed baby greens salad. You can also add already-cooked tiny shrimp to vegetable soup, inside an omelet, or mixed with nonfat mayonnaise and fresh scallions for a "shrimp-salad" sandwich. Try my Shrimp Burrito recipe, a tasty shrimp-rice combo that's sure to please everyone.

## Shrimp Burrito

8 oz. of small precooked shrimp (purchase frozen)

2 cups cooked rice (brown or white)

4 tbsp. green salsa

4 tbsp. reduced-fat ranch salad dressing

1 cup shredded cabbage

4 flour tomato-tortillas

Mix rice, salsa, and dressing together in a bowl. On each tortilla, arrange in the center one-fourth of the rice mixture. Place shrimp (two ounces per tortilla) and shredded cabbage on top. Roll up, folding ends in as you roll. Wrap in foil and heat in a 250-degree oven for 10 to 15 minutes (or use warmed rice, shrimp, and tortillas). Makes four servings.

| **Nutrition Facts** Shrimp Burrito Serving Size 1 | |
|---|---|
| **Amount per Serving** | |
| Calories 406      82 Calories from fat | |
| | % Daily Value |
| Total Fat 9g | 14% |
| Saturated Fat 1g | 6% |
| Cholesterol 111mg | 37% |
| Sodium 496mg | 21% |
| Total Carbohydrate 63g | 21% |
| Dietary Fiber 3g | 11% |
| Protein 19g | |
| Vitamin A 6%   •   Vitamin C 21% Calcium 8%   •   Iron 22% •   Vitamin E 25% | |

# Soybeans (& Soy)

Called the "wonder bean" or "ta-tou," which in Chinese means "greater bean," soy beans are your ticket to heart health. For centuries, soybeans and traditional soybean products, such as tofu and tempeh, have been an integral part of Asian culture—as food, as medicine, and even as a machine lubricant (soybean oil makes a great gear lube). And still today, millions of people in China, Indonesia, and Japan enjoy soy's heart-healing powers. With the Simple Six Eating Plan, you now can experience this wondrous bean and its seemingly magical phytochemicals called *isoflavones.*

For many of you who are soy shy, chowing on a bowl of cooked soybeans may seem a remote possibility, no matter how heart healthy. Does dining on a swishy block of tofu, or nibbling on a soy paste called miso sound a bit too exotic for your taste buds? Perhaps it's not your idea of a delectable way to health, but this versatile bean comes in many variations and forms. I guarantee you there is a soy formulation that you will enjoy and can easily make a part of your daily diet. (You can find out more about the magic of soy in Chapter Two, page 14.)

### Soy Simple

For starters, the nutritional stats on plain old cooked soybeans gives you some indication that this is no ordinary bean. A one-cup cooked serving packs about 25 percent of your daily need for fiber and folate along with a staggering 29 grams of protein, or 50 percent of your daily need. Besides being protein rich, soy protein is superior in quality to other beans and vegetables. In fact, soy protein is similar to the protein in milk and other animal products. And it's the protein in soy that protects your heart. Soybeans also contain about 15 grams of fat per serving, unusually high for a bean. Obviously, that's why soybean oil is a major vegetable oil used in cooking. Perhaps it's alarming that a good-for-you bean is high in fat, but much of this fat is unsaturated, not the cholesterol-clogging saturated type.

Remember from the Simple Six Eating Plan that you are striving for one to two servings of soy foods daily to get 25 grams or more of soy protein daily. Are you thinking what I think you are? "I need to eat a bowl of soybeans every day?" "Is there any other way I can get those 25-plus grams of soy protein I need for heart protection?" Cooked soybeans, which taste surprisingly sweet, almost buttery, are far from the only way to fit the wonders of soy into your life. Adopting soy into your daily fare is easy when you think of soy as a food group rather than a specific food.

A wide array of soy foods awaits you. There are traditional soy foods brought to us from Asian cultures including tofu, tempeh, miso, and natto. "Westernized" or "second generation" soy foods have also made their way onto the scene to accommodate our visual taste for basic foods, including veggie burgers and hot dogs. And to make things even easier, there are now concentrated soy protein powders that you can add to shakes, bread, muffins, and more, and still reap the rewards of soy without even meeting a soybean. All these varieties make soy eating simple.

### Soy Savvy

With the following glossary, you can navigate your way through the many foods made from this ancient healing bean. I list various soy products, where to find them, and the best ways to use them. (Throughout the book, I show more how-to's on tofu and a few other soy foods—see Index.)

- *Tofu*—Made from coagulated soymilk that has been shaped into blocks. Bland tasting, yet it can easily take on desired flavors. Sold fresh in the produce section, in shelf-stable packaging, and also in the freezer section. Use just about any way you want in stir-fries, sauces, dips, desserts, grills, casseroles—think of it as a substitute for eggs, yogurt, and meat.
- *Miso*—A paste made from soybeans that have been fermented with a mold. Often rice or another grain is used in the processing. Found

in grocery stores, Asian food shops, and health food stores. Use as a flavoring in soups, beverages, or as an appetizer.

- *Natto*—Similar to miso with a stronger smell and a cheesy texture. Found in some grocery stores, but more likely in Asian food shops or health food stores. Use as a spread or in soups.

- *Tempeh*—Made from cooked soybeans that are inoculated with a culture to form a dense, chewy texture. Find tempeh in the frozen food section. Use in sandwiches, soups, casseroles, and salads, or try tempeh grilled.

- *Soymilk*—Ground soybeans are mixed with water to form a milk-like beverage. Found in the refrigerated section or in shelf-stable packages in the grocery store. Use as you would milk for drinking, baking, or cooking. Check the label for protein and vitamin mineral fortification. As a milk substitute you want to choose those with added calcium.

- *Soy Flour*—Made from whole soybeans so it contains the same amount of protein, fiber, and fat. You can also get defatted soy flour, which on a weight basis is richer in protein. Find soy flour packaged in your grocery store or sold in bulk in a health food store. Use in baking to replace regular flour. But since there is no gluten (a protein in wheat crucial in raising bread) only replace about 25 percent of regular flour with soy flour when making breads. You can use a bit more when making quick breads, cookies, and muffins. Soy flour tends to brown while cooking so turning down the temperature may be required (best to consult a soy cookbook on more specifics.)

- *Soybeans, fresh or frozen*—Cooked whole beans that you find packaged in the frozen foods section or at times, in the produce section. Use as you would any other beans in salads, casseroles, soups, and more.

- *Soynuts*—Roasted whole soybeans that are either oil or dry roasted. Found in grocery and health food stores. Use as a topping over cereal, yogurt, casseroles, or just as a great snack.

- *Soy Sauce*—Made from ground or whole soybeans, wheat flour, and various fermenting agents. The mixture is then pressed which yields soy sauce. With its strong, salty flavor, this is perhaps our oldest known seasoning. Soy sauce, available at virtually any grocery store, is very low in soy protein and therefore without the heart-healthy isoflavones.

- *Isolated Soy Protein*—Frequently called ISP and made from defatted soy flour, this scoopable powder is very rich in protein. Much of the carbohydrate is also gone so there is no "beany" flavor. This is the soy protein used in a majority of the soy-heart disease research studies. Sold in canisters, you can purchase ISP at some grocery stores or health food stores under the label Health Source® Soy Protein Powder. The company can also be called directly at 1-800-445-3350 (TakeCare®) for mail order. ISP works well as an ingredient in many dishes—casseroles, soups, sauces, pancakes, muffins, cookies, breads, and my favorite—blended drinks. Toss a scoop into your morning fruit smoothie and you have an unbeatable heart-saving drink. Also, look for ISP on the ingredient list of various packaged foods made with soy.

- *Textured Soy Protein*—Made from defatted soy flour that has been pressed giving it a grainy or flaky appearance. You can purchase textured vegetable protein (TVP) in health food stores and in some grocery stores. TVP must be rehydrated with water or vegetable broth for use. Once reconstituted, TVP has a meat-like texture making it a great meal extender in casseroles, tacos, and any dish using ground meat. My favorite TVP use—I rehydrate about a cup with red wine (also heart-smart) and stir into my spaghetti sauce. TVP is also used in ready-to-eat products such as soydogs, burgers, and more.

### *Still More Soy*

If the notion of adding soy to your diet still sounds as far away as its homeland of China and Indonesia, here are a few ways to get you started.

- Stroll the grocery store or health food store for soy products such as breakfast sausages, soydogs, and soyburgers. Pick up one or two new ones each week to try. To get you started, check out the "Veggie Burgers" list; these tasty versions of beef burgers give you a dose of soy goodness.

- Use silken or soft texture tofu in place of yogurt and sour cream.

# Veggie Burgers

Try a faux burger next time you are filling a bun. These patties heat up in a matter of minutes in the microwave, oven, or grill and taste great.

| Brand | Protein Source | Calories | Protein (gm) | Fat (gm) | Fiber (gm) |
|-------|----------------|----------|--------------|----------|------------|
| Morningstar Farms Garden Veggie Patties | Textured vegetable protein, egg whites, brown rice | 100 | 10 | 2.5 | 4 |
| The Original Boca Burger | soy | 84 | 12 | 0 | 5 |
| Ken and Robert's Veggie Burger | organic soybeans, brown rice, Bulgur wheat, soy cheese | 130 | 5 | 1 | 3 |
| Green Giant Harvest Burgers, Original Flavor | soy protein concentrate, isolated soy protein | 140 | 18 | 4 | 5 |

- Try soymilk over your ready-to-eat cereal or hot cereal in the morning.
- Use sliced tempeh for your next sandwich filler.
- Crumble tofu into a spaghetti sauce instead of ground meat.
- Prepare whole, green soybeans as a side dish topped with herbs, or mixed with pasta, chopped onions, and cilantro.
- Reconstitute textured vegetable protein and mix with canned sloppy Joe mix or vegetarian chili.
- And when time is short, for those of you who are a bit timid of tempeh or tofu, use ISP. Whip up a blender drink using Health Source® or another isolated soy protein powder. Combine fruit, ice, fruit juice, and Health Source® for a power shake. Check out my recipe for Midnight Madness on page 82.

## Spaghetti Sauce à la Soy

1 jar ready-to-use spaghetti sauce (no meat added)

1 can ready-cut tomatoes

1 1/2 cups baby carrots, grated or chopped in food processor until fine

1/2 cup red wine

1/2 cup textured vegetable protein

1/2 cup water

2 oz. (or 2 scoops) Health Source® isolated soy protein powder (ISP)

In a large saucepan combine jarred sauce and tomatoes. Bring to a boil and add the grated or finely chopped carrots; let simmer 20 minutes. In a small bowl, combine wine and textured vegetable protein, then add to simmering sauce. Combine water and ISP, stirring to dissolve. Add to simmering sauce, stir completely, and cook another five minutes. Serve over cooked pasta and sprinkle with grated Parmesan cheese. Makes eight servings.

| **Nutrition Facts** | |
|---|---|
| Spaghetti Sauce à la Soy | |
| Serving Size 1/8 recipe | |
| **Amount per Serving** | |
| Calories 189      50 Calories from fat | |
| | **% Daily Value** |
| Total Fat 6g | 9% |
| Saturated Fat <1g | 4% |
| Cholesterol 0mg | 0% |
| Sodium 646mg | 27% |
| Total Carbohydrate 24g | 8% |
| Dietary Fiber 3g | 14% |
| Protein 11g | |
| Vitamin A 91%  •  Vitamin C 39% | |
| Calcium 12%  •  Iron 14% | |
| •  Vitamin E 63% | |

# Spinach

Popeye was right: Spinach is good for you! While Popeye boosted his strength with a can of spinach, this leafy green vegetable actually KO's heart disease and hypertension with a vengeance. A half-cup serving of cooked spinach or about one and a half cups raw contains a staggering quantity of carotenes that help protect artery walls from damage. In addition, a serving of spinach packs a dose of folate which brings down levels of that nasty artery-wrecker homocysteine, and provides the minerals magnesium and potassium to keep hypertension at bay, all in a mere 20 calories.

Spinach contains a mix of carotenes which are plant pigments or colorings that give many vegetables and fruits yellow, orange, and red hues. But spinach is green because of the intense green color of chlorophyll in the leaves that overpowers the orange-yellow color of the carotenes. Despite the camouflage, these carotenes, including hall-of-famer, beta carotene, and two others—lutein and zeaxanthin—all work overtime in protecting your heart.

One serving of cooked spinach supplies about 5 milligrams of beta carotene and over 12 milligrams of lutein and zeaxanthin. Studies show that these carotenes keep circulating LDLs from oxidizing which in turn protects the arteries from these rampaging cholesterol carriers. In one study, women were put on a low carotene diet for a few months and then for about a month took in a mix of carotenes equivalent to a serving of spinach daily. Throughout the study, the researchers sampled the women's LDL levels and tested for how well their diet protected the LDLs from oxidation. Compared to the low-carotene diet, taking in a mix of carotenes protected their LDLs from going "bad."

You can easily reap the benefits of spinach year-round. In your produce section spinach is sold in bunches, as loose leaves (which lessen the waste), or prewashed in sealed bags. The bag version is my personal favorite since I can do a quick rinse before tossing in a salad or stir-fry rather than performing a tedious soaking and rinsing to rid the spinach leaves of grit.

The extra steps required to select and handle fresh greens such as spinach stops a lot of well-minded eaters from munching on these nutritious vegetables.

Here are a few tips to get the most out of your greens.

- Select crisp, firm looking leaves with bright color. Wilted leaves indicate dehydration and age.
- Avoid greens with browned edges or the appearance of rust on the leaves.
- Once you get your greens home, rinse lightly, wrap the base in a paper towel, and place in a plastic produce bag. Store in the refrigerator, preferably in a vegetable crisper. Most greens keep for about five days before wilting (some longer if you change the paper towel and spray lightly with water).
- Before using in salads or other dishes, rinse thoroughly in cold water to clean away grit and dirt (avoid soaking so as not to lose water-soluble nutrients).
- Use a salad spinner or clean towel to dry excess water from greens when making salad.
- For steamed side dishes, or use in soups, stews, and other mixed dishes, chop greens into bigger-than-bite-size pieces (this helps lessen nutrient loss).

Use spinach in tossed salads, as part of the greens mixture or on its own. Spinach's strong flavor goes exceptionally well with citrus wedges (try my Spinach-Orange Salad recipe). Add fresh chopped spinach to soups or stews. I like to add fresh spinach leaves as a layer to lasagna. Add steamed spinach to omelets, frittatas, or alone as a side dish, garnished with fresh herbs and a lemon wedge. You can steam frozen spinach just as well as fresh and not lose out on this leafy green's power-packed nutrition.

## *Spinach-Orange Salad*

1 bag of baby spinach, rinsed well

1 to 1 1/2 oranges, peeled and divided into sections

juice from one lime

2 tsp. olive oil

fresh ground pepper to taste (salt or salt substitute if desired)

1/2 cup roasted almonds, chopped

Toss spinach leaves with orange sections, lime juice, and olive oil. Add pepper (and salt) to taste. Garnish with roasted almonds. Serves six.

| **Nutrition Facts** | |
| :--- | ---: |
| Spinach-Orange Salad | |
| Serving Size 1/6 recipe | |
| **Amount per Serving** | |
| Calories 110      69 Calories from fat | |
| | % Daily Value |
| Total Fat 8g | 12% |
| Saturated Fat 1g | 4% |
| Cholesterol 0mg | 0% |
| Sodium 46mg | 2% |
| Total Carbohydrate 9g | 3% |
| Dietary Fiber 4g | 17% |
| Protein 4g | |
| Vitamin A 44%  •  Vitamin C 61% | |
| Calcium 10%  •  Iron 11% | |
| Folate 32%  •  Vitamin E 47% | |

# Squash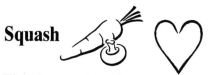

The winter variety of squashes such as butternut and acorn squash (available year-round in your grocer's produce section) come packed with a trio of heart-saving nutrients—beta carotene, vitamin C, and potassium. A half-cup serving of cooked butternut squash supplies over 70 percent of your vitamin A needs as beta carotene, one-quarter of your vitamin C needs, and a hefty 300 milligram dose of potassium. This threesome protects your heart from the damaging effects of cholesterol on your arteries and also helps lower high blood pressure.

Both beta carotene and vitamin C keep the bad cholesterol carrier LDL from going rancid and damaging artery walls. In one study on a group of smokers who notoriously have oxidized or "angry" LDLs as a result of cigarette smoking, a beta carotene rich diet helped to protect the LDLs from oxidizing as readily. This means they are less likely to scar artery walls and deposit vessel-clogging cholesterol. Vitamin C also has the same benefit in protecting against the ravages of oxidized LDLs which is believed to be one of the key steps in the development of heart disease and stroke.

The potassium in winter squash works along with other minerals including calcium and magnesium to help control and normalize blood pressure levels. A serving of winter squash provides about 5 to 10 percent of calcium and magnesium needs. Studies show that individuals who routinely eat diets rich in these three minerals have a lower risk of developing hypertension.

Several varieties of winter squash can be found in the produce section of your local supermarket. Most winter squashes have an inside core of seeds (scoop out before cooking or eating) and flesh that is typically yellow-orange. The most common are:

- Butternut (my favorite), which is club-shaped, peach/pink outer inedible skin (like other winter squashes) and orange inside;
- Acorn, which is green-ribbed and acorn-shaped with orange inside;
- Banana, which is a large squash (sometimes over 20 to 30 pounds—you buy segments of this squash) with orange-yellow inside;
- Hubbard, which is green-ribbed like acorn but much larger in size and pale orange inside;
- Spaghetti, which when cooked comes out as yellow spaghetti-like strands; and
- Turban, which is orange with flecks of red and has a cap-like top.

As long as you store winter squash in a dark, cool, and dry place, they keep for a number of weeks. Winter squash is cooked best by baking in the oven or by microwaving. Cut the squash open and scoop out the seeds. Place face down on a baking sheet (cover surface with foil or spray with canola oil cooking spray) and bake at 300 degrees for about 45 minutes or longer depending on size. The squash's inner flesh should be soft to the poke of a knife. Scoop out the flesh from the outer skin and mix with fresh ground pepper and fresh herbs or top with a sprinkle of maple syrup for a sweet taste. You can also bake squash (acorn is best for this) with fillings of rice, beans, or lean meat. I also like preparing baked squash as I would mashed potatoes. Try my Butternut Squash Casserole for a quick, hearty meal.

### *Butternut Squash Casserole*

1 med. butternut squash, cut in half lengthwise with seeds removed

2 cloves of garlic, crushed

1 small or 1/2 large yellow onion

1 tbsp. olive oil

1/2 cup whole-wheat bread crumbs

1/4 tsp. ground pepper and salt or salt substitute to taste

3 tbsp. grated Parmesan cheese

On a rimmed cookie sheet lined with aluminum foil, place squash cut side down. Bake in a 350-degree oven for 45 minutes to an hour until very soft. Let cool five minutes and scoop out insides, being careful not to include the outer skin, and place in casserole dish (about 3 cups of squash). Sauté garlic and onions in oil and add to squash. Stir in bread crumbs, pepper, and salt. Sprinkle cheese on top and cover dish with foil or lid. Bake at 350 degrees for 10 minutes (longer if ingredients have cooled). Serves six.

| **Nutrition Facts** |  |
| --- | --- |
| Butternut Squash Casserole |  |
| Serving Size 1/6 recipe |  |
| **Amount per Serving** |  |
| Calories 114      33 Calories from fat |  |
|  | % Daily Value |
| Total Fat 4g | 6% |
|    Saturated Fat 1g | 5% |
| Cholesterol 3mg | 1% |
| Sodium 124mg | 5% |
| Total Carbohydrate 19g | 6% |
|    Dietary Fiber 3g | 14% |
| Protein 4g |  |
| Vitamin A 83%   •   Vitamin C 28% | |
| Calcium 10%   •   Iron 6% | |

# Strawberries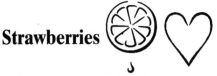

My idea of a fabulous dessert is a bowl of lusciously sweet, fresh strawberries. It's hard to imagine that a fruit that tastes like candy tops the list when it comes to antioxidant power. Recently, a group of researchers from Tufts University in Boston tested strawberries along with 11 other commonly eaten fruits including apples, oranges, and grapes, for their capacity to protect against oxidative damage—the type that can lead to clogged artery walls and heart disease. The number one protector in the group was strawberries.

Strawberries' super-power status comes from an array of goodies, the first of which is vitamin C. About 140 percent of your daily needs are found in a one-cup serving. Strawberries are also loaded with some very special and powerful nonvitamin/mineral substances known as *flavonoids*. Through an almost magical process they act as powerful antioxidants. Strawberries are a particularly good source of two flavonoids called *quercetin* and *kaempferol*. Studies show that these two flavonoids help protect LDLs from oxidizing and becoming dangerous to artery walls. Also, quercetin and kaempferol help keep blood platelets from clumping together, thereby avoiding deadly blood clots and subsequent heart attack or stroke.

Eating a diet plentiful in flavonoids from foods such as strawberries, onions, apples, and tea will help ward off heart disease. That claim is supported by mountains of scientific studies. In fact, one of the largest studies, performed by Researchers from the National Institute of Public Health and Environment Protection in the Netherlands, tracked a group of 800 men 65 to 84 years old for five years, observing their heart health and the number of deaths from heart disease. The scientists also determined flavonoid intake from their diets. Compared to the men who ate the lowest amount of flavonoids, those men who regularly consumed tea, onions, apples, and other flavonoid-rich foods had less than half the risk of dying from heart disease. I'll take those odds any day.

Strawberries can be had year-round from the produce section but their peak (and lowest price) is typically March/April through July. Select strawberries with a full red color, avoiding uncolored or "white" berries or those that are overly seedy. If sold in a sealed plastic container, make sure berries on the bottom are not spoiled or mushy. Always rinse well before eating and avoid letting strawberries sit in water.

Top your morning cereal (hot or cold) with sliced strawberries, or blend a handful into your fruit smoothie. As a snack, try dipping fresh strawberries in vanilla yogurt, or (you have to trust me on this one) dip into a touch of balsamic vinegar and then in brown sugar. Of course, you can add strawberries as a colorful and heart-healthy addition to a fruit salad, or combine with kiwi slices and pineapple chunks on a skewer to make a fruit kabob. While fresh strawberries are often the standard, baked berries are wonderful in a cobbler. Try my recipe topped with a dollop of vanilla yogurt for a sweet strawberry treat.

## Strawberry Cobbler

5 cups cleaned, dehulled strawberries, cut in half

1 tbsp. "sugar in the raw" (light brown sugar crystals)

1 cup flour

3/4 cup brown sugar

1 tsp. baking powder

1 large egg, beaten

1/4 cup butter, melted

Place strawberries in a baking dish, an eight-inch square or round casserole works well. Sprinkle one tablespoon of sugar over the top. Combine flour, baking powder, and sugar in another bowl. Add egg and use a fork to make a crumb mixture. Sprinkle over the top of berries. Drizzle melted butter over the top and bake at 350 degrees for 30 to 40 minutes until top is nicely browned. Makes six servings.

## Nutrition Facts

Strawberry Cobbler

Serving Size 1/6 recipe

| Amount per Serving | |
|---|---|
| Calories 285      81 Calories from fat | |
| | % Daily Value |
| Total Fat 9g | 14% |
| Saturated Fat 5g | 25% |
| Cholesterol 56mg | 19% |
| Sodium 22mg | 1% |
| Total Carbohydrate 50g | 16% |
| Dietary Fiber 4g | 16% |
| Protein 4g | |

Vitamin A 10%   •   Vitamin C 117%
Calcium 5%   •   Iron 13%

# Sunflower Seeds

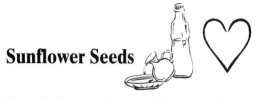

Botanically speaking, sunflower seeds are a fruit. And heart-health speaking, these tiny tidbits are a super-food. Think back to your younger years of munching on roasted sunflower seeds (and spitting out the pieces of shell). You probably didn't realize that you were doing your heart some good. Each one-ounce serving of shelled sunflower seeds contains an almost-unheard-of amount of vitamin E in a single food—140 percent of your needs! And vitamin E literally provides a shield of armor around LDLs, preventing them from becoming oxidized and damaging artery walls.

As LDLs travel through your circulation, they look for places (body cells such as muscle) to drop off their cholesterol passengers. During LDL's travels, oxidative damage may occur which is much like a bus full of passengers careening out of control. The end result (the wreck) is cholesterol passengers (strewn) all over artery walls. Vitamin E protects the LDLs from oxidizing, thereby keeping these cholesterol carriers from spinning out of control and clogging up artery walls.

Studies show that people who routinely eat a diet rich in vitamin E or who take a vitamin E supplement, cut their risk of heart disease. In one study from the University of Minnesota School of Public Health, over 34,000 women were tracked for seven years to investigate vitamin E intake and risk of heart disease. Those women with the highest vitamin E intake from foods had less than half the risk compared to women with the lowest vitamin E intake. Some research studies also suggest that vitamin E keeps heart disease at bay by inhibiting an enzyme involved in the growth of specific smooth muscle cells located in the artery walls which are known to cause heart disease.

Beyond vitamin E, sunflower seeds also provide about a third of your folate needs. Great news, since this B vitamin is needed to help clear the blood factor homocysteine, a normal metabolite that researchers know to be damaging to artery walls in high levels. And while you might cringe at the 14 grams of fat in a serving of sunflower seeds, most of it is polyunsaturated which in most cases is neutral to blood cholesterol levels.

Sunflower seeds are available in their hulls or "hull-less." For snacking, give your mouth a workout and munch on whole sunflower seeds (make sure to spit out the hulls). Sunflower seeds without hulls come in several varieties. Select dry roasted to avoid extra fat. Oil-roasted versions add another two or so grams of fat per serving. If available, reach for no-salt-added sunflower seeds, especially if you've been advised by a physician to cut back on sodium.

Use sunflower seeds as a heart-healthy ingredient in a variety of dishes. Sprinkle on top of your hot cereal, over plain or flavored nonfat yogurt, into a fresh fruit salad or a hearty casserole of rice and beans. I enjoy sunflower seeds as part of a power trail mix that I make up regularly and keep on hand at my desk. Clients seem surprised when I tell them, "This stuff is actually good for you and your heart!" Try it out for yourself!

### *Power Trail Mix*

1 cup roasted, unsalted sunflower seeds

1 cup dried papaya pieces (cut to 1/2-inch size)

3/4 cup white raisins

1/2 cup roasted soy nuts

1 cup oat cereal (Cheerios® or other ready-to-eat brand)

Mix all ingredients together. Store in a tightly sealed container. Makes eight servings.

| **Nutrition Facts** | |
|---|---|
| Power Trail Mix | |
| Serving Size 1/8 recipe | |
| **Amount per Serving** | |
| Calories 264      104 Calories from fat | |
| | % Daily Value |
| Total Fat 12g | 18% |
| Saturated Fat 1g | 5% |
| Cholesterol 0mg | 0% |
| Sodium 36mg | 1% |
| Total Carbohydrate 34g | 11% |
| Dietary Fiber 3g | 12% |
| Protein 10g | |

Vitamin A 30%  •  Vitamin C 39%
Calcium 7%  •  Iron 19%
•  Vitamin E 69%

# Sweet Potato

When Columbus brought back the news to Spain about the New World, he also brought back the North-American native sweet potato. And in no time, this root vegetable became popular throughout Europe. Today we typically serve sweet potatoes during holiday times. (You know, it's that dish made with little marshmallows and brown sugar.) But it's time this member of the potato family makes a regular appearance on your plate. Sweet potatoes are a stellar source of beta carotene. One medium-sized baked sweet potato supplies a staggering 10 milligrams of beta carotene—more than you find in an equal weight of carrots. And that's not all: you get 50 percent of your vitamin C needs, almost 20 percent of fiber, and about 400 milligrams of potassium (same as a small banana) all for 115 calories.

Beta carotene, much like vitamin E, protects the cholesterol-carrying LDLs from oxidative damage, which in turn is bad for your heart and arteries. As an antioxidant, beta carotene can shield the LDLs, preventing them from turning into crazed cholesterol carriers eventually leading to heart disease. One study from the Cardiovascular Research Unit at the University of Edinburgh in the UK found that compared to men with low circulating levels of beta carotene (due to poor intake from vegetables and fruits), the risk of angina or chest pain was less in men with high circulating levels of this antioxidant.

Select and use sweet potatoes as you would white potatoes. Choose potatoes that are firm and without any cut marks or surface injuries. At home, store in a cool, dry place (but not in the refrigerator). Cook sweet potatoes in their skin, which easily comes off after cooking. You can bake, boil, microwave, or even grill sweet potatoes. Add sweet potatoes to stews and soups for a shot of extra beta carotene. Mash with a small amount of low-fat milk or plain yogurt for an incredible side dish. Try my Sweet-Potato Mash made with a touch of garlic and whole-wheat crackers.

### Sweet-Potato Mash

2 large sweet potatoes, cut into 2-inch pieces
1 tbsp. butter
1/4 tsp. garlic powder
fresh ground pepper to taste
8 small whole-wheat crackers

Boil sweet potatoes in a small amount of water until very soft. Drain water and mash well with a fork. Add butter and garlic powder and stir. Crumble wheat crackers and mix into sweet potato mixture. Serve as a side dish with baked fish or chicken. Makes five servings.

| **Nutrition Facts** | |
|---|---|
| Sweet-Potato Mash | |
| Serving Size 1/5 recipe | |
| **Amount per Serving** | |
| Calories 110    30 Calories from fat | |
| | **% Daily Value** |
| Total Fat 3g | 5% |
| Saturated Fat 2g | 8% |
| Cholesterol 6mg | 2% |
| Sodium 43mg | 2% |
| Total Carbohydrate 19g | 6% |
| Dietary Fiber 3g | 10% |
| Protein 2g | |
| Vitamin A 120%  •  Vitamin C 17% | |
| Calcium 1%       •  Iron 3% | |
| •  Vitamin E 28% | |

# Tea

Besides water, tea is by far the world's most popular beverage. Centuries old, tea-drinking is a daily ritual in many countries. Tea often welcomes a guest, serves as a work-break beverage, or as an afternoon spot of relaxation. And making time for tea is good for your heart. New research shows that a special class of phytochemicals called *flavonoids,* found in abundance in tea leaves, helps protect against heart disease and stroke. Whether you like tea green or black, hot or cold, regular or decaf, brewed or instant, sipping on a cup is decidedly a step in the right direction for your heart.

### A Look into Tea Leaves

Both green and black tea are specially prepared leaves picked from the same variety of an evergreen tropical plant. (Herbal teas, which have not been found to have the same health benefits, come from a variety of plants depending on the tea, e.g., peppermint tea.) The only difference between green and black tea stems from the way the tea leaves are prepared after harvesting.

Black tea is made by allowing the freshly picked and chopped leaves to "ferment" or stand for a few hours. This gives the tea leaves time to undergo changes enhanced by a special enzyme. As a result, the leaves turn brownish-black, a variety of flavonoids are formed, and black tea's distinctive taste is born. Green tea is made by first exposing the leaves to heat or hot steam which inactivates the enzyme responsible for turning tea leaves black, hence green tea. The beverage brewed from the green tea leaves is more mild in flavor, but still is loaded with powerful flavonoid phytochemicals.

Besides changing the flavor, the color of the tea has much to do with its heart-protecting powers. About 30 percent of the weight of a dried tea leaf is a type of flavonoid called *catechin.* When the tea leaf remains green, the primary catechin is EGCG (short for *epigallocatechin*). When a tea leaf is allowed to turn black, new catechins called *theaflavins* and *thearubigens* form. Sounds like a chemical brew, but these catechins have powerful antioxidant powers. In fact, research studies show that in a test tube, catechins outpower the notable antioxidants vitamin C and even vitamin E.

The abundance of these catechins in green and black tea gives this beverage a real kick when it comes to heart health.

Catechins help protect the cholesterol-carrying LDLs from becoming "rancid" and infiltrating artery walls causing unwanted fatty buildup. Also, catechins may help prevent blood platelets from clumping together in much the same way aspirin works. Since platelet stickiness can lead to a blood clot—which is a cause for a heart attack or stroke—tea's powers are worth sipping.

### Tea Time

Without a doubt, research studies show that people who drink tea regularly have a lower risk of dying from heart disease. In one study, over 800 men ages 65 to 84 were tracked for their flavonoid intake from tea, onions, apples, and other fruits and vegetables. Those men who consumed the most flavonoids had a lower risk of death from heart disease compared to men with a low flavonoid intake. Over 60 percent of flavonoid intake in all men came from drinking black tea.

Other research shows that when put to the test against other antioxidant-rich fruits and vegetables, tea's catechins outshine the rest. In a laboratory test-tube setup that imitated the oxidation of LDLs in the circulation, tea's catechin, EGCG (in green tea), was found to be 20 times more potent than the well-known antioxidant vitamin C. Catechins in black tea were also found to be potent antioxidants. From the laboratory results, researchers postulate that EGCG and other catechins have a similar impact in the body, protecting LDLs from oxidation. This helps explain why catechins and other flavonoids protect so well against heart disease.

A cup of tea, green or black, has less than half the caffeine of brewed coffee. Those interested in avoiding the caffeine altogether should try decaffeinated tea. In fact, laboratory analysis shows that decaffeinated tea also contains large quantities of those heart-healthy catechins. The decaffeination process carefully removes the caffeine without altering the flavonoid levels. And when tea is poured over ice, catechins are unharmed. Instant tea is made from brewed tea and also contains heart-healthy catechins.

So how many cups of daily tea protect your heart? So far researchers haven't quite pinpointed an exact formula. But in one study a group of healthy volunteers drank five cups of black tea daily for four weeks. The researchers then sampled their blood and isolated the LDLs to see how well they were protected from oxidation. LDLs from the tea drinkers showed much better protection from oxidation than non-tea drinkers. But until more research is done, it's not clear whether a lower daily tea intake would have the same benefits.

Investigations continue to explore the magical powers of tea flavonoids and a specific recommendation on tea drinking may be just around the corner. Until then, we will go with solid science that drinking tea has heart-healthy benefits. It's not clear that taking a tablet that contains tea catechins has the same power. So for now, enjoy tea time—it's good for your heart.

# Tempeh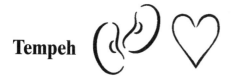

Another in the line of heart-healthy soybean products, tempeh is a must in your Simple Six Eating Plan. Tempeh, which has a nutty, mushroom-like flavor, is made from cooked soybeans that are fermented with an inoculation of a special mold called *Rhizopus oligosporus.* During this process, potent antioxidants form in tempeh which may have heart-disease fighting benefits. Also, tempeh contains the same isoflavones, a class of phytochemicals, found in soybeans which are effective in lowering blood cholesterol levels. And as a result, regular consumption of tempeh, tofu, and other soy products have been shown to help fight off heart disease.

Tempeh was put to the test by researchers from Airlangga University in Indonesia. (By the way, tempeh got its start centuries ago in Indonesia where it is now the most popular soy food.) Seventy-five participants with high levels of blood cholesterol ate either a standard diet or the same diet with the addition of daily tempeh. Following just two weeks on the tempeh-boosted diet, total cholesterol and artery-clogging LDL cholesterol significantly dropped.

In other research, scientists from Japan (another country big into soy products) discovered during the fermentation of tempeh that an antioxidant called *HAA* forms (HAA stands for *3-hydrox-yanthranilic acid,* so I prefer saying HAA). In careful test-tube experiments, HAA acts as a very strong protector against oxidative damage, the same type known to harm LDLs, the carriers of cholesterol that build up on artery walls, and lead to heart disease.

As for its nutritional profile, per half-cup serving tempeh contains 165 calories with six grams of fat, less than a gram of which is saturated fat. Tempeh is also a great source of high-quality protein, about 16 grams per half cup (equivalent to the protein in two eight-ounce glasses of milk.) Tempeh's vitamin and mineral profile is modest with approximately 10 percent of your needs for vitamins $B_6$, $B_{12}$, and folate.

You'll find tempeh in the refrigerator or freezer section of your local grocery store. A few years back, you could only find tempeh in health food stores. But now tempeh is mainstream; and it comes in a variety of tempting flavors—teriyaki, barbecue, and spicy varieties such as Southwest-flavored. Compared to tofu, tempeh is less versatile due to its strong flavor (not to mention tempeh *looks* a bit exotic). In any case, tempeh heated briefly (you can do this in the microwave) makes up into a fabulous sandwich combined with arugula or other greens, red onion, and grilled pepper (if you happen to have these on hand). Tempeh also works well in a stir-fry, Asian-style casserole or crumbled into broth soups. My recipe for soba noodle casserole has an Asian flair and with the cabbage, onions, and ginger combination is a heart-healthy main dish (great for that last-minute potluck obligation).

## *Tempeh-Snow Pea Noodle Salad*

1 package (8 oz.) of soba noodles (buckwheat)

1 8-oz. package of tempeh, diced in small pieces

2 cups of snow peas, cleaned

1 cup of water chestnuts, sliced

1 tsp. sesame oil

1 bunch of scallions, chopped

4 tbsp. light soy sauce (reduced-sodium)

1/4 cup sweet rice wine vinegar

juice of one lime

4 tsp. sesame seeds

Cook soba noodles as directed on package (cook quickly, for about 4 minutes). Rinse noodles when done under cold water and drain. In a large bowl, toss noodles with remaining ingredients. Chill one hour before serving. Makes 5 servings.

## Nutrition Facts
Tempeh-Snow Pea Noodle Salad
Serving Size 1/5 recipe

| Amount per Serving | |
|---|---|
| Calories 322 | 45 Calories from fat |

| | % Daily Value |
|---|---|
| Total Fat 5g | 8% |
|    Saturated Fat <1g | 4% |
| Cholesterol 0mg | 0% |
| Sodium 1121mg | 47% |
| Total Carbohydrate 53g | 18% |
|    Dietary Fiber 5g | 18% |
| Protein 16g | |

| | | |
|---|---|---|
| Vitamin A 1% | • | Vitamin C 69% |
| Calcium 6% | • | Iron 20% |

# Tofu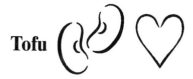

The best known member of the soy family and once the brunt of many jokes, tofu has gained tremendous respect as an exemplary super-food. Tofu is made from soymilk with a coagulant added which forms a curd that can be pressed into cakes. Sometimes called bean curd, tofu has been gracing the plates of millions in

China for some two thousand years. Like its cousins, tempeh and miso, tofu contains powerful phytochemicals called isoflavones that protect your heart. Tofu also supplies a dose of soy protein, shown to help lower cholesterol levels and stave off heart disease.

A four-ounce or half-cup serving of tofu supplies between 13 and 20 grams of soy protein, depending on the texture and type (more on this later). A serving of tofu also packs about 35 milligrams of isoflavones, a daily dose that some researchers feel is helpful in preventing heart disease. There's more to tofu's heart-healthy ingredients. One serving also provides 25 percent of your daily calcium needs. This mineral has been shown to help ward off hypertension.

The isoflavones in tofu are called *genistein* and *diadzein.* These substances protect against heart disease by putting a damper on the cholesterol bad-guys LDLs. In heart disease, during the process of plaque accumulating on artery walls, or what I call sludge buildup, LDLs infiltrate the walls of arteries. When LDLs become damaged or oxidized, they are more inclined to invade artery walls and dump their cholesterol load on your arteries. Also, the size of the LDLs make a difference in the likelihood that they will end up clogging arteries. Big LDLs are more damaging than smaller LDLs.

Studies show that genistein and diadzein protect LDLs from oxidizing which helps keep them from invading and damaging artery walls. Also, new research shows that a diet rich in these isoflavones reduces the size of LDLs, making them less damaging to arteries. And genistein has an additional magical property of keeping blood particles called platelets from clumping and blood from clotting suddenly, which prevent both heart attack and stroke.

Exciting research continues on the powers of isoflavones and more discoveries are right around the corner. Until then, recent studies show that a daily intake of 30 to 50 milligrams of isoflavones may help boost heart health. Tofu and other soy products supply plenty of these isoflavones. A half-cup serving of tempeh, for example, supplies 35 milligrams of isoflavones, as does a serving of tofu. Check the "Isoflavones in Soy" chart for more numbers.

### *For the Tofu Timid*

Looks aren't everything. Lucky for tofu, I kept this in mind years ago the first time I opened up a package. Many of the clients I work with shy away from using tofu on a regular basis not only because of its appearance—a white block of stuff, but also because tofu's looks are intimidating. You're not quite sure what to do with it. Boil? Broil? Bake? Grill? Microwave? And what about the murky water used in packing, should you toss it out? For those of you timid with tofu, and that's just about everyone, here's a primer to put you at ease with this versatile, heart-healthy soy food.

**BUYING TOFU**   You can purchase tofu fresh in the produce section or refrigerator section in your grocery store. It's usually submerged in water. Check the dating on the package. When stored in the fridge unopened, it should last a number of weeks. If opened, change water to help prevent contamination and use within a few days. You can also find tofu in aseptic or shelf-stable packaging. Unopened, this tofu can last at room temperature for up to a year. After opening, store in the refrigerator and use within two days.

Tofu, like regular cheese, comes in different textures and consistencies. Which you choose makes a difference, depending

### Isoflavones* in Soy

| Food | Isoflavones (milligrams per serving) |
|---|---|
| Tempeh, 1/2 cup | 35–40 |
| Tofu, 1/2 cup | 35 |
| Soy Milk, 1 cup | 30 |
| Isolated Soy Protein, 1 oz. | 40–80 |
| Soy Flour, 1/2 cup | 28 |
| Soy links, 1 oz. | 7–15 |

* Isoflavone content in soy foods and soy products varies widely in part due to the actual isoflavone content of soybeans and the measuring techniques.

on how you plan to use the tofu. The texture of tofu is either sponge-like which is referred to as "regular," or custard-like which is called "silken." Each of these two textures comes in three levels of hardness: soft, firm, and extra firm.

When choosing which type of tofu to use, keep in mind that tofu is already cooked. So eating it raw is more than okay; however, you may find that since tofu's taste is quite bland (like noodles), the fun is in combining tofu with your favorite foods. You can use tofu as a substitute for typical foods such as mayonnaise, cheese, eggs, cream, and meats. Or you can use tofu as "is" and view it as an item in your diet rather than a faux replacement for an animal product.

USING TOFU   Regular or silken, soft tofu works well for blending, crumbling, and mashing. Use this tofu in place of cottage cheese, for example, in a lasagna. Or crumbled and then "scrambled" makes a great dish of soy "eggs." Use soft tofu as a base for sauces or dressings. You can even make puddings, pie fillings, and cake "frosting" with soft, silken tofu that has been sweetened.

The firm tofu versions can be cubed and put into salads, soups, stir-fries, or skewered and put on a kebob. Firm tofu also crumbles well and can be put in almost any dish as an accompaniment or complete replacement for ground meat or eggs. Since tofu is already cooked, you can add it during the last few minutes of cooking, in soup for example. If tofu is allowed to cook longer the texture toughens which gives it a more meat-like feel.

Tofu's bland taste lends well to other flavors. In other words, there's no overpowering tofu taste. Tofu takes up other flavors brilliantly; so think marinade. Mix together soy sauce, ground peanuts, and fresh ginger for a tofu marinade. Let tofu sit about an hour or less and then grill, cube into a fresh mixed green salad, or crumble and make exotic scrambled tofu.

TOFU EXTRAS   Products made with tofu such as tofu burgers or baked tofu are also available, usually located in the frozen food section. Simply microwave a minute or two, serve in a whole-grain bun, and you're ready to enjoy a burger that will also make your heart happy. Baked tofu is denser than standard varieties, higher in protein, and typically comes flavored. Usually marinated, baked tofu has a load of sodium so check the label.

## *Tofu à la 'Wave*

(a favorite of mine because it is so easy to make and really tastes great)

1 block of firm tofu (8 oz.)

1 tsp. sesame oil

1/2 cup chopped scallions

1 tsp. sherry

1 clove of garlic, crushed

1 tbsp. pickled ginger, diced

In a microwavable bowl, place the block of tofu. Drizzle the sesame oil and sherry over the top, and then sprinkle the remaining ingredients over the tofu. Cover with plastic wrap and microwave for 45 seconds to 1 minute (depending on microwave power) until the tofu is heated through. Makes two servings.

| **Nutrition Facts** | |
| --- | --- |
| Tofu à la 'Wave | |
| Serving Size 1/2 recipe | |
| Amount per Serving | |
| Calories 122      70 Calories from fat | |
| | % Daily Value |
| Total Fat 8g | 12% |
| Saturated Fat 1g | 6% |
| Cholesterol 0mg | 0% |
| Sodium 77mg | 3% |
| Total Carbohydrate 6g | 2% |
| Dietary Fiber 2g | 8% |
| Protein 10g | |
| Vitamin A 2%    •  Vitamin C 9% | |
| Calcium 14%     •  Iron 36% | |
| •  Vitamin E 51% | |

# Tomato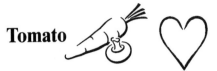

Tops on my list of California-living pleasures is eating vine ripened, juicy tomatoes all summer long. These tomatoes are the real thing—they taste like tomatoes should. I easily consume one to two whole tomatoes daily, and my husband Mark, whose family history puts him at risk for premature heart disease, easily outdoes my tomato intake. I encourage Mark to eat virtually anything made with tomatoes, including processed tomato sauce or juice as a way to lower his risk. The magic heart-disease fighting ingredient in tomatoes is *lycopene.* In similar fashion to other antioxidants, lycopene protects LDLs from becoming dangerous to artery walls and initiating cholesterol buildup.

Like other carotenoids, including beta carotene, lycopene gives fruits and vegetables their wonderful color—in this case, red. (Ruby-red grapefruit and watermelon are also stellar sources of lycopene.) One medium-sized tomato supplies nearly four milligrams of lycopene along with a dose of another antioxidant, vitamin C. The news is even better for tomato-based products. A half-cup of tomato paste that you might add to a pasta sauce or on top of a pizza has a whopping 8.5 milligrams of lycopene. And tomato juice, which you may have avoided because of the sodium, supplies an unbelievable 20 milligrams of lycopene.

According to various research studies, eating a diet rich in lycopene provides protection against heart disease. (Research also points to lycopene as a potent cancer fighter.) In one study, a group of smokers, who notoriously have low circulating levels of lycopene, and nonsmokers were asked to eat a diet high in carotenes, specifically eating more tomatoes.

At the end of two weeks, circulating levels of lycopene and other carotenes improved in both groups. Researchers also sampled the cholesterol-carrying LDLs and tested them for susceptibility to oxidative damage. Following the high-carotene diet, the LDLs in both groups became more resistant to oxidation. This will undoubtedly lower heart-disease risk, particularly good news for smokers who are already at a much greater risk than nonsmokers.

When possible, select vine-ripe tomatoes for eating. Stop at roadside produce stands during the summer months to get your fill. Store tomatoes in a cool place but not a refrigerator, as chilled tomatoes lose their flavor quickly. Out-of-season tomatoes are typically ripened with ethylene gas and as a result lack flavor and often have a crunchy, mealy texture. They also lack the lycopene and vitamin C levels found in vine-ripened varieties. When in doubt about vine-ripe or gassed tomatoes, give them a whiff. Vine-ripe tomatoes have an aromatic tomato odor while the ethylene-gas variety are odorless. Since processed tomato products are more concentrated, they outdo fresh tomatoes when it comes to lycopene. Feel free to use other tomato products like tomato sauce, paste, juice, and catsup.

Tomatoes are tremendously versatile. Used raw, they can invigorate any kind of sandwich, liven up green or pasta salads, and make a wonderful side dish with fresh basil and a touch of garlic and olive oil served over crunchy sourdough bread slices. Try tomatoes chopped raw, or straight from the can in soups, stews, and sauces. My made-from-scratch (instant) spaghetti sauce starts from a ready-to-use jar variety doctored up with ready-cut canned tomatoes, tomato paste, and a touch of red wine—a lycopene powerhouse.

### *Tomatoes Stuffed with Tofu*

4 large tomatoes, washed

2 tsp. olive oil

1/2 yellow onion, diced

1 clove of garlic, crushed

1/2 green pepper, diced

8 oz. of soft tofu, mashed

1/4 cup fresh coriander, chopped

1 tbsp. soy sauce

2 tbsp. grated Parmesan cheese

With a sharp knife, remove the stem end of each tomato. Then scoop out (saving tomato insides), hollowing each tomato leaving about two-thirds of the tomato intact. Sauté onion, garlic, and pepper in oil until soft, then add tomato scoopings and sauté another two minutes. In a bowl, mix together tofu, coriander, and soy sauce; then add tomato mixture. Generously fill each tomato with this mixture and arrange in a baking dish. Sprinkle cheese on top of each and bake at 375 degrees for about 20 to 25 minutes.

## Nutrition Facts

Tomatoes Stuffed with Tofu

Serving Size 1 stuffed tomato

| Amount per Serving | |
| --- | --- |
| Calories 113      54 Calories from fat | |
| | % Daily Value |
| Total Fat 6g | 10% |
| Saturated Fat 1g | 7% |
| Cholesterol 2mg | 1% |
| Sodium 331mg | 14% |
| Total Carbohydrate 9g | 3% |
| Dietary Fiber 3g | 10% |
| Protein 7g | |

| Vitamin A 11% | • | Vitamin C 55% |
| --- | --- | --- |
| Calcium 11% | • | Iron 21% |

# Tuna

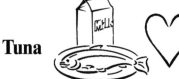

In the U.S., canned tuna ranks number one in the seafood category. Both canned and fresh tuna also rank on top of the chart of heart protectors. Tuna comes with disease fighting omega-3 fats, which cut the risk of suffering from a heart attack. A 3-ounce serving of grilled, fresh tuna supplies almost two grams of omega-3s and is also a fabulous source of protein—half your daily need. Tuna also supplies a staggering amount of vitamin $B_{12}$, which works with other B vitamins including folate to clear excess circulating homocysteine. This amino-acid metabolite is a key suspect in the development of heart disease.

The threat of a sudden heart attack is greatly reduced with more omega-3s—more fish in your diet. These special fats reduce the "stickiness" or "clumping" of platelets, the substance in the blood responsible for clotting. A sudden blood clot formed in the coronary arteries or brain can bring on a heart attack or stroke.

To test the "anticlumping" ability of omega-3s, researchers from the University of Western Australia in Perth studied a group of 120 men at risk for heart disease due to their elevated blood pressure and circulating cholesterol levels. The men were asked to take either fish oil capsules containing omega-3s or eat more fish in their diet over a 12-week period. Compared to pretreatment, both fish oil capsules and fish in the diet reduced platelet "clumpability." This helps explain why regular fish eaters have a lower risk of suffering from a sudden heart attack.

Whether fresh or canned, tuna makes a great addition to your Simple Six Eating Plan. If buying fresh tuna, make sure fish has been properly stored on ice in the market and use it the day you bring it home. Grilled or baked tuna first marinated in a simple lemon-juice/soy-sauce marinade (add a sprig of fresh herbs) makes a fabulous main meal served with a mixed green salad and seasoned polenta or rice.

Canned tuna speaks for itself—it's easy to keep on hand, simple to open, and usable in scads of ways. Purchase the water-packed variety to save on added fat from the oil. And select a low-sodium version if you've been advised to cut back on sodium (one serving of regular water-packed tuna has over 300 milligrams of sodium). Use chilled tuna in green salads, pasta salads, or serve as an appetizer on top of small bread rounds with a sprig of watercress or coriander. Still my favorite ways to use canned tuna are in tuna-salad sandwiches and tuna-noodle casserole. When making tuna salad, liven up the tuna with fresh dill, finely chopped celery, and nonfat mayonnaise. Here's my tuna-noodle casserole recipe with a secret touch of oat bran, for a dose of cholesterol-blasting fiber.

## *Tuna Salad with a Twist*

2 cans of tuna, white meat packed in water

1 12-oz. bag of Rotelle pasta (twisted or corkscrew shape), cooked as directed, drained

1 red onion, chopped

1/2 cup fresh basil, chopped

1 tbsp. olive oil

1/2 cup black olives, sliced

1/4 cup capers

juice from 2 limes

4 large tomatoes, chopped

fresh ground pepper to taste

In a large bowl, mix cooked, drained pasta with remaining ingredients. Chill for at least an hour before serving. Best served over a bed of fresh romaine lettuce. Makes eight servings.

| **Nutrition Facts** | |
|---|---|
| Tuna Salad with a Twist | |
| Serving Size 1/8 recipe | |
| **Amount per Serving** | |
| Calories 282        36 Calories from fat | |
| | % Daily Value |
| Total Fat 4g | 6% |
| Saturated Fat <1g | 2% |
| Cholesterol 7mg | 2% |
| Sodium 246mg | 10% |
| Total Carbohydrate 42g | 14% |
| Dietary Fiber 2g | 7% |
| Protein 18g | |
| Vitamin A 8%  •  Vitamin C 24% | |
| Calcium 7%  •  Iron 16% | |

# Turkey

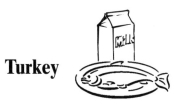

Once just relegated to the Thanksgiving dinner table, turkey is making inroads onto dinner plates year-round. Turkey makes a great fit in the Simple Six Eating Plan. But let's talk turkey. Many people I work with on their eating plans believe that switching to ground turkey from beef makes all the heart-healthy difference in the world.

That's not exactly true. Turkey, especially turkey products such as sausage, hot dogs, and ground turkey, may not be the nutritional dream food you thought. But with a bit of label reading savvy and some turkey sense, you can make turkey a part of your healthy menu plan. Straight, unadulterated roasted turkey (without the skin) is good stuff. It's a great source of protein, with 25 grams or half your daily need in a three-ounce serving of either light or dark meat. Fat content is higher in dark meat compared to white: six grams in dark versus three grams in white meat. Turkey is also a good source of the minerals iron (more in dark meat), zinc, and copper.

But ground turkey is a different story when it comes to fat. Most ground turkey brands include white and dark meat along with fat-laden skin. This explains why a three-ounce serving of ground turkey contains almost 11 grams of fat, and three grams of it are artery-clogging saturated fat. When shopping for ground turkey, take a good look at the Nutrition Facts food label. Purchase brands that are 97 to 99 percent fat-free which means about three grams of fat or less per serving.

As for turkey sausage, bacon, or hot dogs, check the food labels. Some versions can be as loaded down with fat as traditional versions. Compare the number of grams of fat in a serving to your daily fat budget from the Simple Six Eating Plan. (Note the serving sizes too, as you may unknowingly be eating two plus servings at a time.) Since about a third of the fat in many processed turkey products is saturated, use caution. It's best to reserve these products for special occasions or just make sure turkey dogs are not one of your daily dietary staples.

If day-long cooking, basting, and all-around hassle comes when you think turkey, think again. You can now purchase pre-cooked turkey roasts, which contain both light and dark meat, that can be heated up in a matter of minutes. Serve with mixed greens, steamed vegetables, and boiled red potatoes for a hearty meal. You can use leftover turkey in salads, sandwiches, casseroles, soups, and even stews. I like to open a can of ready-to-eat soup or reduced-fat canned stew, heat, and then stir in leftover turkey meat.

### *Turkey and Yogurt Curry*

1 large turkey breast (1 to 1 1/2 pounds), skin removed and sliced into pieces the size of a quarter

8 oz. of low-fat plain yogurt

1 yellow onion, chopped

5 cloves of garlic, chopped

1 tsp. fresh ginger, chopped

1 tsp. red chili pepper, chopped fine

1 tsp. coriander

1 tsp. cumin

1 tsp. turmeric

2 cloves

1 cinnamon bark

3 tbsp. olive oil

2 cups of frozen (or fresh) peas

Sauté onions, ginger, red chilies, and remaining spices in oil over medium heat in a large skillet. Add turkey and sauté another three to four minutes. Add yogurt and one cup of water, cover, and simmer approximately 20 to 30 minutes until meat is done. Add peas and heat through. Serve over rice. Makes five servings.

| Nutrition Facts | |
|---|---|
| Turkey and Yogurt Curry | |
| Serving Size 1/5 recipe | |

| Amount per Serving | |
|---|---|
| Calories 292      90 Calories from fat | |

| | % Daily Value |
|---|---|
| Total Fat 10g | 16% |
| Saturated Fat 2g | 10% |
| Cholesterol 81mg | 27% |
| Sodium 140mg | 6% |
| Total Carbohydrate 16g | 5% |
| Dietary Fiber 3g | 13% |
| Protein 34g | |

| Vitamin A 8% | • Vitamin C 21% |
|---|---|
| Calcium 13% | • Iron 17% |
| | • Vitamin $B_6$ 34% |

# Walnuts

The Romans knew a good thing when they had it in the palm of their hands. They named the walnut in honor of their god and king, Jupiter. Little did the Romans know, however, that their favorite nut works wonders for the heart. Despite walnuts' high fat content, studies show that eating this nut daily actually leads to a drop in cholesterol levels. A one-ounce serving contains 180 calories and a hefty 18 grams of fat. But the fat in walnuts is far from dangerous. Unlike other vegetable oils (with the exception of flax seed—see page 142), walnuts have a fair amount of omega-3s— the famous fats known to help protect against heart disease.

Dr. Joan Sabaté and other researchers from Loma Linda University in California put daily walnut eating to the test in a group of healthy men with normal levels of blood cholesterol. The men ate three servings of walnuts each day for four weeks. And to keep fat intake steady, the men cut back on other sources of fat in the diet such as margarine and salad dressings. At the end of the test period, the men experienced a 12 percent drop in total cholesterol levels and a 16 percent drop in the cholesterol bad guys, LDLs. And more good news, the ratio of LDL to HDL (good cholesterol carriers) dropped which translates to a lower risk for heart disease.

Speculating on how walnuts work, Dr. Sabaté's group suggested that the profile of fats in walnuts (low saturated and more polyunsaturated) may benefit the heart. Substituting walnut oil, usually available in the cooking oil section of your grocery store, for other fats in the diet such as margarine, may also help lower cholesterol levels. Check the Simple Six Eating Plan for how much oil and other fats to use in your daily fare (Chapter Two, see page 22).

The time of year for walnuts is the fall. I know this only too well as I have the fortune of riding my bike regularly through majestic walnut orchards in California. Fresh, shelled walnuts have that wonderful crunch, but you can get packaged walnuts anytime of year. To help preserve their omega-3 fats, store walnuts well sealed in the refrigerator or freezer.

Walnuts blend well with other flavors in food. Walnuts and chocolate (chocolate chip cookies with walnuts, for example) come to mind as a dynamo combination, but there are others. Cheese and walnuts, mixed greens and walnuts, fruit and walnuts, and cooked grains and walnuts all make fabulous taste combinations. Put chopped walnuts on top of your morning cereal, or toast a handful in the oven and sprinkle into a mixed green or a fruit salad. Pears and walnuts were meant for each other. Try out my salad recipe; the low-fat goat cheese adds to the taste and provides a kick of calcium to boot.

### *Pear-Walnut Salad*

3 ripe pears
1/2 cup walnut halves
2 oz. plain goat cheese, crumbled into dime-size pieces
1 tbsp. lemon juice

Slice pears into thin strips and place in bowl. Put walnuts on a small cookie sheet and bake in a 350-degree oven for 7 to 10 minutes, until nuts are slightly browned. Let cool slightly and toss with pears and crumbled goat cheese. Makes four servings.

## Nutrition Facts
Pear-Walnut Salad
Serving Size 1/4 recipe

| Amount per Serving | |
|---|---|
| Calories 175     87 Calories from fat | |
| | % Daily Value |
| Total Fat 10g | 15% |
|    Saturated Fat 2g | 9% |
| Cholesterol 3mg | 1% |
| Sodium 67mg | 3% |
| Total Carbohydrate 21g | 7% |
|    Dietary Fiber 4g | 15% |
| Protein 3g | |

| | |
|---|---|
| Vitamin A 0% | • Vitamin C 12% |
| Calcium 3% | • Iron 3% |
| | • Vitamin E 11% |

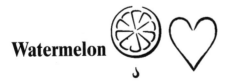

# Watermelon

This sunshine fruit of summer has a rather modest nutrition profile—a sprinkling of fiber, potassium, and vitamin C. But when it comes to warding off heart disease, watermelon packs a punch that's hidden in its rich red color. Lycopene, a member of the carotene family (the most famous being beta carotene), gives watermelon its brilliant color as well as its heart-disease fighting power. As an antioxidant, lycopene helps protect the LDLs from oxidizing, which means stopping the first step in the development of heart disease.

A one-cup serving of watermelon supplies a whopping 6.6 milligrams of lycopene in just 50 calories. Once in the body, lycopene finds its way to parts of the body where fat is located such as fat cells and lipoproteins, namely LDLs, the primary carriers of cholesterol in the circulation. Here lycopene protects against oxidation, which is caused by normal metabolism as well as oxidants such as cigarette smoke and air pollutants. With lycopene and other antioxidants such as vitamin E shielding LDLs from damage, heart disease can be thwarted.

Researchers from various parts of the world including Germany, Finland, and the U.S. studied the relationship between lycopene levels in the body and risk for heart disease. Researchers sampled the lycopene levels in fat tissue in over 1000 men and found that in men with higher lycopene levels, risk for heart disease was about half that of men with low lycopene levels. This translates to eating a diet richer in lycopene (found also in guava, red grapefruits, and tomato and tomato products) to decrease your risk for heart disease.

Make the most out of summertime by eating watermelon often. When buying a whole watermelon, select one that is free of deep pits or cut marks. And there is a reason for knocking on a watermelon to see if it's ripe. A ripe watermelon gives a muffled or dull sounding "ping" while an unripe melon gives a higher pitched sound when knocked with a finger or two. If you're buying precut watermelon, make sure the texture does not look mealy or pithy and that there are no white streaks in the flesh.

Eating watermelon plain (and spitting the seeds across the lawn or out the window) is perhaps the most satisfying way to embrace this fruit's goodness. You can also cut watermelon into bite-size chunks for a fruit salad or add onto a fruit kabob skewer. Blend watermelon chunks (less the seeds) into your blender along with other fruits for a super, heart-healthy smoothie. Try my tropical smoothie recipe with a kick of soy.

## *Tropical Blender Blast*

1 cup watermelon without seeds

1/2 papaya

1 oz. isolated soy powder, vanilla flavored

1/2 banana

1/2 cup nonfat milk or soy milk

5 ice cubes

2 tsp. honey

Place all ingredients in a blender and blend on high until well mixed. Serve immediately. Makes one serving.

| **Nutrition Facts** | |
| --- | --- |
| Tropical Blender Blast | |
| Serving Size 1 | |
| **Amount per Serving** | |
| Calories 342      31 Calories from fat | |
| | % Daily Value |
| Total Fat 3g | 5% |
| Saturated Fat 0g | 0% |
| Cholesterol 0mg | 0% |
| Sodium 258mg | 11% |
| Total Carbohydrate 67g | 22% |
| Dietary Fiber 6g | 25% |
| Protein 17g | |
| Vitamin A 33%  •  Vitamin C 30% | |
| Calcium 26%  •  Iron 28% | |
| Vitamin $B_6$ 52%  •  Folate 39% | |

# Wheat Germ

Wheat germ has long had the image of a true "health" food, and for good reason. As the portion of a wheat kernel that turns into a seedling or new plant, wheat germ is a stellar source of heart-healthy nutrients such as vitamin E and folate. Wheat germ also supplies a dose of vitamin $B_6$, potassium, and fiber. This combination of nutrients may work together in your battle against heart disease and studies show that adding wheat germ to the diet helps lower blood cholesterol.

A one-quarter cup serving of wheat germ supplies 40 percent of your daily vitamin E needs (recall that vitamin E protects the bad carrier of cholesterol—LDLs—from becoming oxidized and damaging artery walls). Each serving also supplies 50 percent of folate needs. This B vitamin helps normalize circulating levels of homocysteine, a protein-like substance in the circulation known to contribute to heart-disease risk.

Adding wheat germ to your daily diet may be an effective way to help lower blood cholesterol and lower heart-disease risk. Scientists from the National Institute of Health and Medical Research Unit in Marseille, France, put wheat germ to the test in a group of people with high levels of blood cholesterol. For 14 weeks the subjects ate about an ounce of wheat germ (one-quarter cup) daily while eating a standard diet that was not low in fat, about 40 percent of the total calories.

The daily dose of wheat germ resulted in a significant drop in the participant's cholesterol levels. And more good news, the LDL level dropped even more. Researchers are not clear what substance in wheat germ is responsible for such dramatic results. But for right now, it is important to know that making a place for wheat germ in your diet will have a double impact on your heart-disease risk by lowering both cholesterol and LDL levels.

Wheat germ, sold in jars or small cardboard boxes, is usually located in the breakfast cereal aisle. Skip the wheat germ versions with added sugar or honey; you are better off getting pure wheat germ goodness. While wheat germ is nutrient rich, it contains a small amount of polyunsaturated fats which can easily break down and spoil. Because of this, you should refrigerate wheat germ once you open the package (wheat germ keeps about five to six months in the refrigerator).

View wheat germ as a food "booster." Sprinkle a few tablespoons over your hot or cold cereal. Try topping yogurt or applesauce with the nutty crunch of wheat germ. Or throw into a fruit smoothie for a heart-healthy boost. Use wheat germ as an ingredient in baked or cooked foods. Add to muffins, pancakes, casseroles, meatloaf, and even brownies. Check out my wheat-germ brownie recipe, it's my favorite and was a secret until now!

### *Fudgy Wheat-Germ Brownies*

1 6-oz. package semisweet chocolate chips

3 tbsp. butter

3/4 cup quick cooking oats

1/3 cup toasted wheat germ (no sugar added)

1/3 cup nonfat dry milk powder

1/2 tsp. baking powder

1/2 cup chopped walnuts

4 egg whites

1/2 cup brown sugar (packed)

1 tsp. vanilla

In a microwave-safe dish, melt chocolate chips and butter at 80 percent power (takes 45 seconds or so depending on the microwave). Blend well and set aside. Combine dry ingredients in a bowl. In another large bowl, beat egg whites with sugar and vanilla until slightly thick. Stir in chocolate ingredient and then dry ingredients; blend well but do not overmix. Spread in 8 x 8 x 2-inch baking dish sprayed with cooking spray. Bake 20 to 35 minutes in a 350-degree oven until edges are firm and top is crisp. Cool completely before cutting or refrigerate overnight before serving. Makes 12 servings.

| **Nutrition Facts** Fudgy Wheat-Germ Brownies Serving Size 1 brownie | |
|---|---|
| Amount per Serving | |
| Calories 221     105 Calories from fat | |
| | % Daily Value |
| Total Fat 12g | 18% |
| Saturated Fat 5g | 25% |
| Cholesterol 9mg | 2% |
| Sodium 57mg | 2% |
| Total Carbohydrate 26g | 9% |
| Dietary Fiber 2g | 8% |
| Protein 6g | |
| Vitamin A 8%     •     Vitamin C 1% Calcium 9%     •     Iron 8% | |

# Wine

No one knows for sure who was the first to make wine. But some 8,000 to 10,000 years ago, an unknowing soul accidentally let the juice of a sweet fruit—perhaps dates, figs, or even grapes—ferment. The outcome: The sugar in the juice fermented to alcohol and wine was born. Since that first jug, wine has been, and is today, a staple beverage of many cultures. In Mediterranean countries, for example, people sip wine daily at meals, and it's believed to be one of the reasons heart-disease rates are low in this European region.

The notion that wine may be good for you is not new. Hippocrates, the father of medicine, referred to wine's attributes in his writings. And today, we know from many research studies that people who drink wine in moderation—that is, one or two glasses daily with meals—have lower death rates from heart disease and stroke.

### *Taking Wine to Heart*

Wine's health benefits appear to be twofold. The alcohol in wine, whether red or white, helps protect the heart; and the phytochemicals from the skins of grapes that end up in wine, especially red varieties, also provide protection from heart disease. These two "attributes" raise wine above other alcoholic beverages as a good-for-you beverage. But as with anything, especially alcoholic beverages, moderation is key. In this case, more is definitely not better.

Scientific studies show that moderate drinking of alcoholic beverages in both men and women lowers heart-disease risk. Alcohol protects your heart by increasing the number of HDLs. These cholesterol-carriers act like good guys by scavenging loose cholesterol and bringing it back to the liver for eventual excretion from the body. Compared to teetotalers, moderate drinkers tend to have greater HDL levels and lower heart-disease rates.

Beyond alcohol, wine provides other heart-healthy benefits. Grape skins contain a class of phytochemical called *flavonoids*. When red wine is made, the juice ferments with the skins allowing the flavonoids to leach into the wine. This process imparts both flavor and color to the wine. As a result, red wine contains flavonoids. (Grape skins are removed during the making of white wines, hence a very low flavonoid content.) These flavonoids, primarily quercetin, help take care of your heart by protecting your LDLs and preventing dangerous blood clots. (Red or purple grape juice also contains flavonoids but only about one-quarter to one-third the concentration found in red wine.)

Studies show quercetin may protect the LDLs, cholesterol bad-guys, from oxidizing and furthering damage to artery walls. In one study, participants drank red wine daily and their blood was sampled to isolate the LDLs. Under laboratory conditions, the LDL taken from the wine-drinking participants was less inclined to oxidize or "go bad" compared to that from non-wine drinkers. Also, research from the University of Wisconsin shows that red wine flavonoids also help keep the blood platelets from becoming sticky. This means blood clots are less likely to form, lessening a chance of a heart attack.

The heart-healthy benefit of wine, primarily red wine, should be put in perspective. Studies that confirm red wine is good for the heart also reveal that those people also typically consume their wine with meals. Therefore, the timing and amount may be crucial in how both alcohol and flavonoids impact heart health. In fact, in regions of Italy and France where heart disease is low, moderate wine drinking is learned from an early age around the dinner table. Displays of drunkenness are virtually nonexistent, and finding pleasure in sipping wine slowly at meals is the cultural norm.

As I tell my patients, drinking an entire bottle one night and then dividing this by seven for a "moderate" average over the week is missing the point. The key here is moderation at all times. I suggest, if wine is an item you would like to include on a regular basis, that you enjoy wine for the pleasure of the palate and the way it complements the many flavors in your meals.

### A Word to the Wise Before You Drink to Your Heart's Content

Before you rush out and buy a bottle of vino, proceed with caution. Alcohol consumption, and this includes red wine, is not without risks.

- Heavy drinkers (4 to 5 drinks or more per day) have a greater risk of developing hypertension. This increases the chance of stroke and kidney failure. Heavy drinking also increases the likelihood of liver damage.

- For women, the increased risk of cancer (particularly breast cancer) with drinking must be weighed with the potential benefit of lowering heart-disease risk. Talk over your cancer risk with your physician before you decide on moderate alcohol consumption (one drink per day).

- Alcohol consumption increases the risk of injuries and accidents at work and on the roadway.

- Heavy drinking also causes liver damage and liver disease.

- Regular drinking may also impair mental function and memory.

## What's a Drink?

The U.S. Department of Agriculture defines moderate drinking (based on research) as:

1 or fewer drinks per day for women

2 or fewer drinks per day for men

One drink equals:

12 ounces of beer (150 calories, on average)

5 ounces of wine (100 calories)

1.5 ounces of 80-proof distilled spirits (e.g., vodka) (100 calories)

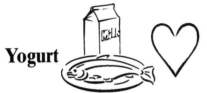

# Yogurt

Yogurt, like cheese and beer, is one of those ancient foods that most likely was stumbled upon. If you leave milk out on a hot day, you get yogurt—fermented milk that has coagulated into a pudding-like, smooth-textured soup. Yogurt has long been noted for its health benefits such as boosting the immune system and perhaps, though not proven, extending longevity. And yogurt, along with small amounts of cheese, is the primary dairy staple among people eating a traditional Mediterranean diet noted for its heart-protecting powers. While researchers are not clear as to how, yogurt appears to boost your heart health by steadying blood pressure levels and keeping cholesterol levels in check.

A one-cup serving of nonfat plain yogurt with just over 100 calories supplies a staggering 40 percent of your calcium needs. A low-fat yogurt, with only 140 calories per cup, also supplies this much calcium. Fruit flavored yogurt (fruit-on-the-bottom style or pre-stirred) is lower in calcium because some of the space is taken up by the added fruit and sugar. Plain yogurt is also rich in the mineral potassium. Both of these minerals play a major role in normalizing blood pressure.

Many studies show that people who eat a diet that meets or exceeds the requirements for these minerals are likely to have healthy blood pressure readings. In one study involving over 52,000 female nurses, those women with a low intake of calcium had a greater risk for developing hypertension. And since many women fall short on meeting their calcium needs, yogurt makes a heart-smart addition to a woman's diet.

Yogurt as part of your daily fare may also provide some benefit to blood cholesterol levels. In a study conducted at University of California at Davis, by Drs. Christine Trapp and Carl Keen, a group of senior adults ages 55 to 70 were instructed to eat a cup of yogurt daily for four months. Compared to another group who abstained from daily yogurt, blood cholesterol and LDLs stayed steady, while they rose in the no-yogurt group.

Purchase yogurt that is either nonfat or low-fat rather than whole milk yogurt that has almost five grams of saturated fat. You are better off selecting plain yogurt and then adding your own flavoring such as fresh fruit, nuts, or wheat germ rather than yogurt with added fruit and sugar that, as I mentioned, is somewhat lower in calcium because there is less actual yogurt per serving. Also look for yogurts that contain live or active cultures. This means the helpful bacteria is still "living" and when eaten has potential health benefits.

You can use yogurt in so many ways. Think of it as a replacement for mayonnaise or sour cream. In this way, use yogurt in salad dressings, sandwich spreads, pasta salads, and potato salad as well as dips for fresh vegetables. Yogurt also works well in making "cream" soups (add at the end of cooking just enough to heat through). Yogurt also works well in curries (see my Turkey and Yogurt Curry recipe on page 282). I give my mashed potatoes a tangy, creamy flare by stirring in a cup of nonfat, plain yogurt instead of milk during mashing.

Yogurt is a standard ingredient in smoothies. It gives a creamy texture without the fat. Of course, eating yogurt as is, topped with fresh fruit and a drizzle of honey, makes for a cool snack. Or try yogurt covered with fresh chopped vegetables and herbs for a new taste sensation. Here's a recipe for a great spinach dip. I usually make this before dinner and let friends and family munch away dipping veggies while we put together the main course.

## *Spinach-Yogurt Dip*

2 cups nonfat plain yogurt

1 10-oz. package of frozen spinach, thawed and drained

1/4 cup reduced-fat ranch dressing

1 tsp. dry mustard

1 8-oz. can of water chestnuts, sliced and then cut into slivers

3 scallion spears, chopped

fresh ground pepper to taste

Mix yogurt, dressing, and mustard together in a bowl. Add the other ingredients and stir. Refrigerate 30 minutes for flavor to "settle." Serve with raw vegetables (cucumber slices, baby carrots, radishes) or triangle-shaped wedges of pita bread. Makes 10 to 12 servings.

### Nutrition Facts

Spinach-Yogurt Dip

Serving Size 1/10 recipe

| Amount per Serving | |
|---|---|
| Calories 60 | 0 Calories from fat |

| | % Daily Value |
|---|---|
| Total Fat 0g | 0% |
| Saturated Fat 0g | 0% |
| Cholesterol 0mg | 0% |
| Sodium 113mg | 5% |
| Total Carbohydrate 11g | 4% |
| Dietary Fiber 2g | 6% |
| Protein 4g | |

| Vitamin A 22% | • | Vitamin C 17% |
|---|---|---|
| Calcium 12% | • | Iron 6% |

# Zucchini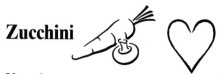

If you've ever grown your own vegetables (or known a neighbor with a vegetable garden) you most certainly had more zucchini than you knew what to do with. This member of the summer squash family makes a great addition to your Simple Six Eating Plan. Loaded with potassium and with only 15 calories per half cup cooked, you can't go wrong with zucchini (no matter how much you have!).

In the now famous clinical trial, Dietary Approaches to Stop Hypertension, or DASH, researchers put study participants on an eight-week program that included eating 8 to 10 servings of vegetables and fruits daily. This amount is twice current recommendations set forth in the Dietary Guidelines for Americans and the Food Guide Pyramid (that triangle-shaped eating guide often seen on food packages). Compared to another group of participants eating a typical American diet, blood pressure, both systolic and diastolic, dropped significantly. In fact, the vegetable-fruit charged diet led to a drop in blood pressure equal to that seen with medications. Great news if you like zucchini and other vegetables and fruits.

How vegetables, such as zucchini, and fruits help lower blood pressure is most likely a combination of reasons. Potassium along with another mineral, magnesium, found in vegetables and fruits both play a role in controlling blood pressure. Also the fiber in fruits and vegetables (zucchini supplies two grams per half cup—almost 10 percent of needs) has been shown to help lower blood pressure, perhaps in combination with other nutrients in these foods.

Zucchini is readily available year-round in your local supermarket's produce section (unless of course, you have a vegetable garden). Select small to medium-sized zucchini, from a few inches to eight inches long. Larger zucchini (and they can get a few feet long) have a mealy, almost woody texture, and are less tender than smaller versions.

Small zucchini are best in stir-fries, added to soups, grated in muffins and breads, or in stews and casseroles. You can also grill zucchini by blanching (place in boiling water for a few minutes) then marinating and tossing onto the hot grill. This makes a great addition to grilled fish or tofu. Larger zucchini are better suited for baking with a stuffing of rice and mushrooms or another favorite concoction. This soup recipe (adapted from *Tofu Cookery* by Louise Hagler, a must cookbook for the tofu timid) uses lots of zucchini and incorporates tofu to boot!

### *"Zufu" Soup*

1 1/2 lb. of small to medium length zucchini, sliced

1 yellow onion, chopped

3 cloves of garlic, crushed

1 tbsp. olive oil

2 cans vegetable stock

1/4 tsp. fresh ground pepper

1/2 tsp. dill

8 oz. of soft tofu, blended in food processor with 2 tbsp. soymilk or skim milk

In a soup pot, sauté zucchini, onion, and garlic in oil. Add vegetable stock and seasonings. Cover and simmer 20 minutes. Add blended tofu and heat through. Serves six to eight. (Great with whole-wheat sourdough bread.)

| **Nutrition Facts** | |
| --- | --- |
| "Zufu" Soup | |
| Serving Size 1 cup | |
| Amount per Serving | |
| Calories 88 | 43 Calories from fat |
| | % Daily Value |
| Total Fat 5g | 7% |
| Saturated Fat <1g | 3% |
| Cholesterol 0mg | 0% |
| Sodium 301mg | 13% |
| Total Carbohydrate 8g | 3% |
| Dietary Fiber 2g | 8% |
| Protein 5g | |

| | | |
| --- | --- | --- |
| Vitamin A 7% | • | Vitamin C 21% |
| Calcium 6% | • | Iron 15% |
| | • | Vitamin E 21% |

# *Index*

*Page numbers in italics refer to tables.*